Economic Impact of Worksite Health Promotion

Joseph P. Opatz, PhD

St. Cloud State University, St. Cloud, Minnesota

Editor

A publication of the
Association for Worksite Health Promotion

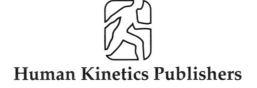

Human Kinetics Publishers

Library of Congress Cataloging-in-Publication Data

Economic impact of worksite health promotion / Joseph P. Opatz, editor;
  Association for Worksite Health Promotion.
     p.   cm.
  Includes bibliographical references and index.
  ISBN 0-87322-436-1
  1. Health promotion--Economic aspects.   2. Industrial hygiene.
  I. Opatz, Joseph P.   II. Association for Worksite Health Promotion.
  RC969.H43E26   1994
  658.3'82--dc20   93-19102
                                                              CIP

ISBN: 0-87322-436-1

Copyright © 1994 by the Association for Worksite Health Promotion

Photo Credits: Pages 1, 143, and 193: The Travelers Taking Care Program; Page 121:
Courtesy of The Travelers; Pages 33 and 67: Photograph courtesy of AENHANCE®
Aetna Life & Casualty's Health Enhancement Program; Pages 51 and 177: File
photos—Wellness South, Inc.; Pages 65, 99, 159, and 209: Johnson & Johnson
Health Management, Inc.; Page 145: © Beebe/Custom Medical Stock Photo

Acquisitions Editor: Richard D. Frey, PhD; Developmental Editor: Julia Anderson;
Assistant Editors: Sally Howe, Julie Lancaster, Lisa Sotirelis, John Wentworth,
and Valerie Hall; Copyeditor: Dianna Matlosz; Proofreaders: Kathy Bennett and
Holly Gilly; Indexer: Barbara Cohen; Production Director: Ernie Noa; Typesetting
and Text Layout: Sandra Meier; Text Design: Keith Blomberg; Cover Design: Jack
Davis; Interior Art: Jim Hampton; Printer: Braun-Brumfield

Printed in the United States of America   10 9 8 7 6 5 4 3 2 1

Human Kinetics Publishers
Box 5076, Champaign, IL 61825-5076
1-800-747-4457

Canada: Human Kinetics Publishers, Box 24040, Windsor, ON N8Y 4Y9
1-800-465-7301 (in Canada only)

Europe: Human Kinetics Publishers (Europe) Ltd., P.O. Box IW14,
Leeds LS16 6TR, England
0532-781708

Australia: Human Kinetics Publishers, P.O. Box 80, Kingswood 5062,
South Australia
618-374-0433

New Zealand: Human Kinetics Publishers, P.O. Box 105-231, Auckland 1
(09) 309-2259

Contents

Part III   Worksite Health Promotion Profiles   143

Preface

I recall in the early 1980s fielding a question from a member of the audience to which I was presenting one of my first talks on wellness. The questioner wanted to know whether the wellness movement was emerging as a long-term trend or was just another fad. I responded that wellness promotion was here to stay, the necessary outcome of a number of factors that were leading business, industry, and government toward a more rational approach to disease prevention and control of health care costs. But I must admit that my private convictions on the subject may have been somewhat less certain than my public response. We had so little information at that time on which to base predictions.

In the interim, the landscape of health promotion has become much more detailed and well understood. The effectiveness of worksite health promotion and the concomitant pressures brought on by ever-increasing health care costs have continued to broaden our role in discussions about better management of health care dollars and improvement in quality of life. This book is another step in a continuing process to illuminate the types of worksite interventions that can lead to improved productivity and reduced benefit outlays. The purpose is to provide a compendium of empirical and theoretical papers on important issues relating to the economic impact of worksite health promotion. Too often readers must rely on scattered sources for the most up-to-date information on this important subject. Although we cannot include all important research being done, by having major studies representing a breadth of subject matters at their fingertips, readers can easily familiarize themselves with current information.

Economic Impact of Worksite Health Promotion is intended for a wide audience of professionals, including those representing the health fields, fitness centers, corporate health promotion programs, human resource and personnel departments, and universities. It is also a useful text for the increasing number of courses, both graduate and undergraduate, that focus on worksite health promotion.

The book is organized into three parts. Part I, "Economics and Worksite Health Promotion," includes three chapters that address some of the important theoretical considerations affecting worksite health promotion. These include the process of creating programs that will have a positive economic impact, problems in trying to measure the costs and the benefits of health promotion, and the benefits resulting from such programs. This part comprehensively reviews the history of worksite health promotion programs and the role that health care costs have played in their development.

Part II, "Assessment and Evaluation," details considerations and techniques for properly evaluating worksite health promotion programs. Chapters 4 to 6 explore the effectiveness of health promotion in reducing health risk and define program evaluation, going through each stage of effective evaluation. The authors explain how to use data commonly available to business, such as insurance claims and information from employee surveys, to measure program effectiveness.

Part III, "Worksite Health Promotion Profiles," looks at programs within specific worksites and at specific program components, featuring both private industry and the public sector. The programs profiled are mammography screening at a large corporation, Morgan Guaranty Trust; risk-rated benefits as implemented by a medium-sized company, Foldcraft Corporation (Kenyon, Minnesota); cost-containment strategy for employees of the local government in Birmingham, Alabama; health promotion for public school employees in the Hurst-Euless-Bedford Independent School District (Texas); and the comprehensive LIVE FOR LIFE program at the Johnson & Johnson Corporation.

And, finally, the appendix presents a white paper prepared for the Association for Worksite Health Promotion 2 years ago. This paper provides a useful overview of the field of the economic impact of worksite health promotion as well as a comprehensive reference list.

This publication is part of the continuing effort of the Association for Worksite Health Promotion (formerly the Association for Fitness in Business) to be the leader in providing the latest information on the economic impact of worksite health promotion programs. The association is the preeminent international organization in this area; it integrates, unifies, and serves a variety of interdisciplinary professionals for the purpose of influencing corporate decision-makers in the areas of health promotion, disease prevention, and health care cost management. In many ways the Association for Worksite Health Promotion establishes the standard for health promotion programming and professional practice at the worksite. I would like to thank the board of directors of the association, and in particular Dr. Robert Kaman, the past president, for their strong support of this publication.

Joseph P. Opatz

PART I

Economics and Worksite Health Promotion

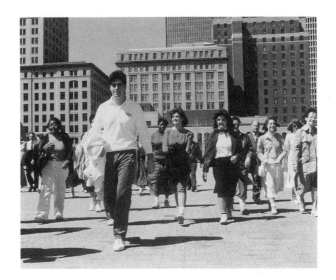

The past 10 years have been a period of rapid growth and change for the field of worksite health promotion. In Part I, three chapters provide different perspectives on the application of economic models to the worksite health promotion industry. Chapter 1, by Chris Lovato, Lawrence Green, and Gene Stainbrook, reviews the history and current state of the worksite health promotion field and was prepared with grant support from the National Institutes of Health and the National Institute for Occupational Safety and Health. It offers a thorough explanation of how the field has developed over the past 4 decades and the role that the costs of health care have played in its growth.

Chapter 2, by David Chenoweth, uses profiles of three companies representing small, medium, and large organizations to relate the general principles of worksite health promotion economics to specific real-world examples. Some of the practical problems and implications of identifying the costs and benefits of worksite health promotion are delineated.

1

The complexity and difficulty of using health costs as a reasonable indicator of health status can make the task of specifying the economic impact of a particular worksite health promotion program difficult. In chapter 3, Wendy Lynch addresses some of the hazards of making the economic case for worksite health promotion and cautions about problems of methodology and interpretation of findings.

Chapter 1

The Benefits Anticipated by Industry in Supporting Health Promotion Programs in the Worksite

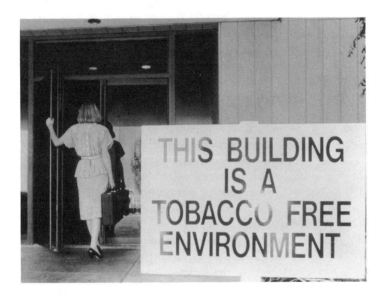

Chris Y. Lovato
Lawrence W. Green
Gene L. Stainbrook

In this review we examine the growth of the worksite health promotion movement, assess the rationale and experience behind three examples of programs adopted by industry, and attempt to account for the diffusion and incorporation of programs among employers.

The Upsurge of Health Promotion Programs

American business and industry took a fresh look at disease prevention and health promotion in the late 1970s as they faced alarming increases in the cost of medical care and health insurance. These costs, falling increasingly heavily on employers, eroded the negotiable benefits for employees and placed a financial strain on many businesses. Emerging research also provided a clearer picture of the sources of medical service cost increases. Several government documents published both in Canada and in the U.S. summarized many of the major research findings and provided guidelines for subsequent policy and program development.

Broad policy statements on the causes of death and status of health of populations were published in two Canadian reports (Laframboise, 1973; Lalonde, 1974). The second of them, commonly referred to as "The Lalonde Report," led to immediate policy initiatives in Canada and had a sizeable spillover effect in the United States. Much of the conceptual and empirical work that formed the basis of the Lalonde report developed in the U.S., but the U.S. government had not put the pieces together in the form of a policy platform. The Canadian report provided a stimulus and a framework for U.S. government attention to these issues.

Lalonde used Laframboise's concept of the health field to describe the major determinants of health and disease and, therefore, the major targets of health promotion and disease prevention. In this framework, it was proposed that the state of human health was a function of four major classes of factors: human biology, health care organization, environment, and lifestyle. The critical discussion of the relative importance of the four categories had a notable impact on the perception of priorities.

In the years preceding the Lalonde report, reductionistic tendencies in medical research were matched by the practice of medicine with more and more specialized, technology-dependent, and impersonal methods and organizations. Thus, both medical research and practice were highly concentrated in the human biology and health care organization categories. This progressive hypertrophy and the consequent atrophy of environmental and behavioral concerns had many critics. Nevertheless, the trends were tacitly accepted by government, the public, and the medical profession.

Some critics, however, were not only outspoken but also articulate and literary. Rene Dubos's *Mirage of Health* (1959) provided a broad sociobiological analysis of the misplaced emphasis. Thomas McKeown's (1971) *A Historical Appraisal of the Medical Task* addressed many of the major issues covered by Dubos and added a critique of medical research and organized medicine. Ivan Illich's (1976) *Medical Nemesis* launched a series of critiques against both the research establishment and organized medicine. A collection of critical essays by health experts in *Doing Better and*

Feeling Worse: Health in the U.S. (Knowles, 1977) also was influential. Several books about the "self-care" and "wellness" movements further fueled the shift in emphasis (Ardell, 1979; Caplan & Killilea, 1976; Levin, Katz, & Holst, 1976; Pelletier, 1979).

Other publications have more directly influenced the increased interest in disease prevention and health promotion programs in business and industry. A widely circulated report by the National Chamber Foundation (1978) on the need for American businesses to take a more active role in the containment of medical costs and in disease prevention was influential. An article in the report exhorted businesses to get actively involved in health education and health promotion for employees and their families (Sehnert & Tillotson, 1978). Subsequent reports on preventive medicine and health promotion sponsored by the Health Insurance Association of America and specific segments of the industry were a further stimulus to program development (Berry, 1981; Kotz & Fielding, 1980; McNerney, 1980).

Some U.S. government reports were influential in stimulating greater general interest in health education and health promotion (U.S. Department of Health and Human Services [USDHHS], 1979a, 1980). Foremost among those directed at work settings were the *Proceedings of the National Conference on Health Promotion Programs in Occupational Settings*, sponsored by the Office of Health Information, Health Promotion, Physical Fitness and Sports Medicine (USDHHS, 1979b). The background papers for this report were published in 1980 in a special issue of *Public Health Reports* on health promotion at the worksite. A subsequent committee co-sponsored by the same office and the National Center for Health Education produced guidelines for management and evaluation of worksite health promotion programs (Parkinson et al., 1982). In 1984, *Prospects for a Healthier America* (USDHHS) outlined objectives and strategies for health promotion in business and industry, reflecting public and private sector consensus.

Two criteria, epidemiological importance and the demonstrated effectiveness of interventions, were used by the Public Health Service to establish the national priorities in health promotion outlined in *Health Objectives for 1990* (USDHHS, 1990). These priority areas included reduction of smoking, reduction of alcohol and drug misuse, diet and nutrition, physical fitness and exercise, and stress management. Other priorities involving behavior and lifestyle, such as injury control and hypertension control, fell under the rubrics of health protection and preventive health services.

In 1991 the Department of Health and Human Services released *Healthy People 2000: National Health Promotion and Disease Prevention Objectives* (USDHHS, 1991). This report details measurable goals and programs targeted for the year 2000 in the areas of health promotion, health protection, preventive services, and surveillance and data systems. The objectives are based on the input and extensive involvement of government, professional organizations, businesses, and individual citizens in a nation-wide effort that involved more than 10,000 people. Priority areas include physical activity and fitness, nutrition, tobacco use, and alcohol and other drugs.

The health priorities and objectives for the nation are intended not merely as a set of federal objectives but also as a basis for state and local government and private sector action (Green, 1980; McGinnis, 1982). Indeed, attainment of the objectives will require the involvement of community-wide efforts that include worksites, elementary and second-ary schools, college campuses, medical care settings, churches, and community organizations. The national priorities provide a general framework, but most organizations will set their own priorities in the context of their particular needs, demands, and resources. The private sector objectives and priorities will be recast from such perspectives as optimum productivity for business or continued revenues for clinics and hospitals.

Setting Priorities Among Worksite Health Promotion Options

Various criteria have been used by organizations to set priorities in health promotion and disease prevention. The more commonly cited criteria are listed in Figure 1.1. These are not necessarily representative of all pro-grams, only of published accounts.

When organizations consider their own needs, resources, and potential benefits, different priorities tend to be established. When immediate costs from poor employee morale, absenteeism, low productivity, and injuries are considered, reduction of alcohol abuse often is given top priority and physical activity and preventive mental health services are moved into second place. When employee interests and company image are primary concerns, fitness facilities or programs are often given a high profile.

- Cost-benefit and cost-effectiveness considerations
- Prior demonstration of benefits in comparable sites
- Time frame for the realization of benefits
- Relevance of the program to health costs and risks in the company
- Employee interest in the program
- Possible negative effects of the program

Figure 1.1   Criteria used in setting health promotion priorities as reported in published accounts of programs in the workplace.

Rationale for Health Promotion Programs in the Workplace

One reason for the choice of worksites as settings for health promotion programs relates to demographics. In 1988, males accounted for an esti-mated 55% of the United States work force and females accounted for

45% (U.S. Department of Labor [USDL], 1992). Demographic data suggest that the work force of the future will be older and include more women and minorities. In addition, the number of new workers joining the work force will decline.

Males are at greater risk for injuries, premature disability, and death from most chronic diseases than are females. Men typically have been harder to reach through traditional medical care and public health programs and are less likely to use preventive physical and mental health services (Cataldo, Herd, Green, Parkinson, & Goldbeck,1986; Kizer, 1987). Females, nevertheless, represent an increasing proportion of the work force, a proportion projected to exceed 60% by the 21st century (USDL, 1992). Women also have caught up with men on some risk factors, such as smoking, which predisposes them to increasing incidence of future chronic disease (USDHHS, 1990).

The growing ethnic diversity of the U.S. population will continue to be reflected in the makeup of the work force. African Americans currently make up 12% of the U.S. population and are the largest minority, Hispanics represent 8% of the population, the second largest minority group, and Asian Americans represent the third largest minority population. These populations are extremely heterogeneous, and the variations within each group are great. For example, the Hispanic population includes Mexicans, Puerto Ricans, Cubans, and other peoples of Central and South American origin. The challenge for employers will be planning and delivering health promotion programs that take into account the needs of these diverse ethnic groups (Aguirre-Molina & Molina, 1990). Similar to the U.S. male population, these populations have been more difficult to reach through traditional medical care and public health programs. Health promotion can play a significant role in addressing the health needs of these groups through programs that are offered in the workplace.

Besides the demographic factors, work settings have logistical, professional, and scientific advantages for health program development and delivery. These advantages include greater access to adults than other community programs; reasonable stability of the target population; organizational structures and management to support the programs; ability to provide preventive medical services at lower costs; and opportunities to develop and provide more comprehensive, integrated health programs than possible through traditional medical care and public health institutions.

Within its broad organizational framework, business and industry can provide a full spectrum of services from prevention and early detection to referral and treatment. For example, in the case of alcohol and other substance abuse problems, employers can use deterioration of job performance to detect problems and to encourage the employee to seek early intervention.

Worksites provide a setting for the development of health-related or behavior-related interest groups and social support networks among employees. Also, if cost-benefit and cost-effectiveness studies are important, worksite-based programs can provide data with known parameters and can facilitate tracking individuals over time.

It is difficult for traditional medical care and public health institutions to provide such a comprehensive and integrated set of preventive medical services. Thus, the work setting represents the single most important channel through which a large proportion of the adult population can be reached systematically through health information and health promotion programs.

Surveys of Worksite Health Promotion Programs

Over the past 20 years, worksite programs have become much more common. Surveys indicate progressive increases in the variety and number of health promotion programs offered in work settings since the mid-1970s (Davis, Rosenberg, Iverson, Vernon, & Bauer, 1984; Fielding & Breslow, 1983; Fielding & Piserchia, 1989; Kiefhaber, Weinberg, & Goldbeck, 1979; USDHHS, 1987). A survey comparing health promotion programs offered by community providers in four midwestern U.S. cities found that worksites provided 40% of all programs offered to adults (Weisbrod, Pirie, Bracht, & Elstun, 1991).

In 1979, the Washington Business Group for Health (WBGH) sponsored a survey that indicated that over 50% of the companies responding offered some form of health promotion program (Kiefhaber et al., 1979). This report described basic health issues of concern to business and industry and highlighted the activities of progressive, successful companies. Though the survey was limited to WBGH members (primarily Fortune 500 companies) and the response rate was only 37%, the report created a sense of awareness and competition among other corporations. Many either issued detailed reports on their own health education and health promotion programs or initiated new programs (Parkinson et al., 1982).

In a survey of California businesses with 100 or more employees, Fielding and Breslow (1983) found that over 75% offered one or more health promotion activities. Nearly two thirds of the company programs, however, were limited to two or fewer activities. The programs ranged from relatively brief, inexpensive cardiopulmonary resuscitation (CPR) seminars to more detailed and expensive hypertension screening and control programs and exercise facilities.

A survey of Colorado businesses with 50 or more employees indicated that approximately 25% offered one or more preventive services on a regular basis (Davis et al., 1984). In addition, 50% of the companies surveyed expressed interest in developing a program. Overall, it was estimated that fewer than 5% of employers in Colorado offered programs on an ongoing basis. This figure was close to the estimated 2% to 5% of employers nationwide who offered ongoing health promotion programs (Warner & Murt, 1984).

The American Hospital Association's 1984 survey of all community hospitals and short-term federal general hospitals, with a response rate of 59%, found that 33% of the hospitals offered health education and health promotion programs to corporate business clients. These programs included CPR (34%), stress management (22%), smoking cessation (22%), weight control (17%), and various others (Ross et al., 1985).

A survey of worksite health education and health promotion programs sponsored by the U.S. Department of Health and Human Services in 1986 found that nearly two thirds of all worksites having 50 or more employees had programs of some kind. Table 1.1 shows the relative prevalence of the types of programs.

In addition to survey results, there are less direct indicators of an increase in the number of disease prevention and health promotion programs at worksites. The growth of professional and commercial organizations also reflects the rising level of activity. Cunningham (1982) reported that the Association for Worksite Health Promotion grew from 25 members in 1975 to over 3,000 in 1981. The increase in the number of business coalitions and the active involvement of more than 50% of them in health education and health promotion services is another indicator of the expansion of the field (Yenny & Behrens, 1984). The large increase in the number of articles on health promotion and worksite wellness programs in both

Table 1.1
Most Frequently Cited Categories of Worksite Health Promotion Activities

Program	Prevalence (%)
Smoking control	35.6
Health risk assessment	29.5
Back problem prevention and care	28.5
Stress management	26.6
Exercise and fitness	22.1
Off-the-job accident prevention	19.8
Nutrition education	16.8
Blood pressure control	16.5
Weight control	14.7

Note. From "Frequency of Worksite Health Promotion Activities" by J. Fielding and P. Piserchia, 1989, *American Journal of Public Health,* **79**(1), pp. 16-20. Copyright 1989 by American Public Health Association. Adapted by permission.

the lay press and in professional journals reflects increases in both interest and, to some extent, program activity (Ardell, 1984; Bibeau, Mullen, McLeroy, Green, & Foshee, 1988; McLeroy, Green, Mullen, & Foshee, 1984; Ware, 1982).

The number and variety of future worksite health promotion programs is also increasing steadily. Many more companies appear to be poised to start new programs or are interested in obtaining technical assistance and support to begin programs. Small companies present the most difficult challenge to community organizations that seek to expand services to employees.

Benefits of Specific Programs

Smoking control, alcohol abuse detection and referral for treatment, and physical activity programs are examples of worksite health promotion efforts commonly supported by employers. Though individual program areas are described for the purposes of this chapter, it is important to note that single-focus, one-shot programs cannot realistically reduce health care costs or accrue other benefits, such as reduced absenteeism, increased productivity, and long-term behavior change related to health risks.

Smoking Control

Smokers have a 70% greater overall mortality rate for disease than do nonsmokers. Almost 400,000 deaths occur each year from the effects of cigarette smoking (USDHHS, 1989a). In principle, the extremely strong association between smoking and four of the leading causes of death and disability, namely cancer, heart disease, stroke, and chronic obstructive lung disease, should give antismoking programs a prominent place in work settings. The increased risk of lung cancer, heart disease, and other smoking-related diseases results in higher insurance rates for smokers. Therefore, companies that promote smoking cessation programs could benefit by reduced group insurance premiums. Unfortunately, high mobility and turnover of the labor force, as well as the relatively long time required for smoking to produce notable economic consequences related to chronic diseases, make smoking prevention and cessation programs appear less attractive to companies as a cost-containment strategy (Kristein, 1983). In some cases, economic conflicts of interest (such as advertising revenue from tobacco companies) may dampen the will for a strong antismoking policy (Kiefhaber & Goldbeck, 1984; Warner, 1987).

A stronger case for smoking cessation programs in most companies can be made when more immediate costs associated with smoking are considered. These costs include time lost to smoking rituals, extra clean-up costs, damage to furniture and equipment, and inefficiencies and errors related to factors such as high carbon monoxide levels, eye irritation, and sickness while on the job, which also can lead to absenteeism and lost productivity. One smoker can cost a company an estimated $336 to $601 a year (Kristein, 1983).

Smoking has negative effects not only on smokers but also on non-smokers. Environmental tobacco smoke released into the air as a result of tobacco smoking is a hazard for nonsmokers. There are more than 1,200 potentially toxic chemicals in tobacco smoke. Many of these substances are released in sufficient quantity to pose health risks through the burning of only a few cigarettes (American Lung Association, 1982). Recent reviews of the effects of passive smoke have concluded that the adverse effect of second-hand smoke both on individuals with preexisting health conditions and those in good health is sufficiently documented for business and industry to regulate smoking at the workplace (Eriksen, 1986; Eriksen, LeMaistre, & Newell, 1988; Fielding, 1991; USDHHS, 1986).

Smoking will be implicated increasingly in liability and compensation claims associated with occupational illnesses, because of its interaction with and potentiation of other worksite hazards. This trend will continue stimulating insurance carriers to pressure industries to control smoking, unions to pressure members to reduce smoking so that management cannot use employee smoking as a basis to avoid liability for occupational hazards, and employees to pressure employers to restrict smoking in work areas and thus reduce the risks of second-hand smoke.

Nonsmoking Policies.   In addition to the many smoking cessation efforts aimed at individuals, strict bans on smoking are becoming increasingly common. In a national survey of worksites with 50 or more people, 27% reported having a formal smoking policy (Fielding, 1990). Surveys in Massachusetts and California indicate that approximately 50% of companies had such policies in the late 1970s and early 1980s (Bennett & Levy, 1980; Fielding & Breslow, 1983). Legislative, judicial, and administrative decisions at the federal, state, and local levels have combined to increase the interest and involvement of employers in controlling smoking at the workplace (Eriksen, 1986; Gottlieb, Eriksen, Lovato, Weinstein, & Green, 1990; Shimp, 1978). Other factors that have stimulated corporate programs include initiatives or requests from occupational health staff, health departments, voluntary agencies, research scientists, and employees themselves (Vojtecky, Kar, & Cox, 1985). By the late 1980s, the prevalence of such written policies approached 50% (Gottlieb et al., 1990). In 1990, the U.S. Environmental Protection Agency classified environmental tobacco smoke as a known human carcinogen, thus adding both support and incentive for employers to initiate nonsmoking policies.

Legal avenues used successfully by nonsmokers to restrict smoking at worksites include appeals to the employer's duty to provide a safe, healthful work environment and the high cost of disability payments, retirement benefits, workers' compensation, and unemployment compensation (Walsh & Gordon, 1986). A key strategy has been the use of appeals for protection from wrongful discharge or other retaliation by employers because of an employee's protest against worksite smoking and for protection under the Rehabilitation Act of 1973, which requires reasonable accommodation due to a handicap (e.g., hypersensitivity to tobacco smoke). However, ". . . no constitutional right to a smoke free environment has been established, although attempts have been made by the First, Fifth, Ninth and Fourteenth Amendments" (Eriksen, 1986, p. 81).

It is unclear whether restrictive smoking policies are associated with reductions of cigarettes smoked per individual (Fielding, 1991). These environmental controls seem only to shift smoking activity to nonwork time (Carey & Abrams, 1980; Gottlieb et al., 1990; USDHHS, 1986).

Smoking Cessation Programs.   At Control Data Corporation, current smokers and smokers who had quit less than 5 years earlier generated 25% more benefit payments and twice the number of hospital days than those who either never smoked or quit more than 5 years earlier. Smokers who enrolled in smoking cessation courses sponsored by Control Data Corporation smoked an average of 1.6 packs a day at the start of the course. Twelve months after the course, 30.3% were not smoking, 43.5% were smoking less than one pack a day, and 24.2% were smoking one or more packs a day (Naditch, 1984).

Under the Johnson & Johnson LIVE FOR LIFE program (see chapter 11), a company-wide smoking cessation program produced significant reductions in the number of employees who smoked. Results of a 2-year study indicated that 22.6% of all smokers in the comprehensive wellness program quit smoking versus 17.4% of smokers in a comparison group that received health screening only (Shipley et al., 1988).

A study to evaluate the relative effectiveness and cost-effectiveness of self-help and group methods of smoking cessation for employees found that the quit rate for the two groups was 17% at 18 months. Although the cost for each participant was twice as high for the clinical (i.e., group) approach as for the self-help kit ($32 vs. $16), the cost for each successful quitter was similar in both groups ($150). The authors recommended that employers offer a choice of these two methods in order to attract the largest number of participants possible (Bertera, Oehl, & Telepchak, 1990).

In a review of 21 formal, quantitative evaluations of worksite smoking cessation programs (Bibeau et al., 1988) extending the earlier reviews of Danaher (1982), Orleans and Shipley (1982), and Windsor and Bartlett (1984), 15 studies depended on pre-experimental designs (posttest only, or pretest and posttest, with no comparison group), 3 used quasi-experimental designs (nonequivalent comparison group), and 4 used true experimental designs with equivalent control groups. Smoking quit rates for these worksite-based programs were comparable to those of clinical programs, however, posttest follow-up was limited.

Worksite smoking cessation and control programs have taken varied forms ranging from clinical and self-help behavioral models to organizational, regulatory, and legal reform of smoking policies. Results have been at least as good as those of programs in clinical settings, but the benefits to employers who sponsor the programs remain largely conjectural. Generally, studies suggest that more intensive programs using multiple sessions and multiple components have higher success rates than shorter term, less intensive interventions.

Alcohol Abuse Detection and Treatment

The National Council on Alcoholism reports that 1 in 10 employees has a serious problem with alcohol. Alcohol abuse influences the health and welfare of employees, families, and employers (Cook & Youngblood, 1990; National Institute on Alcohol Abuse and Alcoholism, 1984).

Approximately 50% of all motor vehicle injuries are alcohol related. Many nonwork injuries are also linked to alcohol use. Up to 57% of all industrial injuries are associated with alcohol, and as high as 75% of those employees who have been involved in two or more industrial accidents have alcohol problems (Berry, 1981). Alcohol also contributes to the high costs of psychosocial disturbances and domestic violence that accrue to industry health care plans. Approximately 65% of all affective disorders, 40% of all crime, 87% of all homicides, 50% of all child abuse cases (probably more of spouse abuse), and up to 84% of suicides are associated with alcohol abuse (Giesbrecht et al., 1988; Roizen, 1982; USDHHS, 1989b). Productivity is compromised by alcohol problems. Unemployment, often a secondary consequence of alcohol abuse, has tremendous spin-offs in many costly ways.

Employee Assistance Programs.   In the 1940s, only a few companies had industrial alcoholism programs (Dunkin, 1982). Increasingly, as private and public organizations began to acknowledge the high costs associated with alcohol abuse, many took steps to prevent or minimize them. Among the approaches taken by employers to reduce alcohol-related costs were educational activities, training management to identify problems, referral, self-help groups for alcoholic employees, and employee assistance programs (EAPs).

EAPs often have been an outgrowth of alcoholism detection and treatment programs. In contrast to most alcohol treatment programs, the functions of some EAPs span the continuum from primary prevention to treatment and rehabilitation. Thus, many EAPs have expanded their focus beyond crisis intervention and treatment to include a variety of more preventive services (Brody, 1988; Walsh & Kelleher, 1987).

Comprehensive EAPs address employees' mental and emotional problems that interfere with work performance and could develop into more serious and costly psychiatric or physical disorders. A major purpose of many current programs is to assist employees in solving work-related problems *and* problems outside work that compromise work performance and quality of life. A wide range of job-related, family-related, legal, financial, mental and emotional, and substance abuse problems are addressed by EAPs (Klarreich, Francek, & Moore, 1985; Spicer, 1987). More recently, EAPs have begun to take an active role in AIDS prevention and education (Bunker, Eriksen, & Kinsey, 1987).

Initially, most preventive services were provided on a one-to-one basis or in a counselor-patient mode. In some newer programs, training in time management, stress management, and personal finances are being offered in small group or even classroom formats. Evidence of the acceptance and success of this progression from treatment services to prevention and education is important for several reasons. First, it suggests a greater awareness on the part of employees of the nature of their problems and an increased willingness to take the initiative in solving them. Second, it shows that some preventive mental health services can be made convenient and cost-effective in the context of work settings. Third, it suggests that even those preventive mental health services coordinated by employers and made conveniently available outside the workplace may help reduce the incidence of mental illness and work performance problems.

Many companies now offer in-house EAPs or contract out for these services. Results from the National Survey of Worksite Health Promotion Activities (USDHHS, 1987) indicate that 52% of worksites with 750 or more employees offered an EAP. The structure and function of the EAPs varied with the companies. Some used in-house staff exclusively; others contracted with vendors for services; some did both.

In larger organizations, small in-house staffs, usually counselors or social workers, were employed on a full- or part-time basis to provide brief therapy or to refer employees to outside services (Backer, 1987). The size of a company is strongly related to its likelihood of providing an EAP. Fielding and Piserchia (1989) found that 52% of worksites with 750 or more employees had EAPs, whereas only 15% of worksites with 50 to 99 employees had EAPs.

Many businesses have found that company-sponsored EAPs pay for themselves and often result in cost savings. EAPs have been reported to reduce absenteeism, injuries, and medical utilization. A major reason for the increased interest in and expansion of these programs has been their reported potential to contain and reduce health-related costs.

General Motors Corporation has developed a comprehensive EAP that provides services at over 130 sites to an estimated 7%, or over 44,000, of their North American employees. After the first year of their program, General Motors reported a 40% decrease in lost time, a 60% decrease in sickness and accident benefits, a 50% decrease in grievances, and a 50% decrease in on-the-job accidents (Berry, 1981).

Major commercial insurance carriers in the United States have estimated that about $5 are ultimately saved for each $1 spent in alcohol rehabilitation efforts (Dupont & Basen, 1982). General Motors estimated a 3-to-1 return on dollars invested in their employee assistance program, Equitable Life Assurance Company estimated 5.5-to-1, and Kennicott Copper, a slightly higher return of 6-to-1. Overall these results indicate favorable cost-benefit ratios for programs designed to help employees to resolve both on- and off-the-job problems. Though these results are very promising, few studies have been rigorously evaluated, and good long-term cost-effectiveness studies are needed (Kurtz, Googins, & Howard, 1984).

The development of improved surveillance of alcohol-related problems and the provision of accessible, acceptable preventive and treatment services have shown promising results. Still, even though seeking assistance for alcohol and other substance abuse-related problems has become more acceptable, many employees enter alcohol or drug treatment programs only because their supervisors requested they do so, usually after detecting a serious decline in work performance. Entering and completing a substance abuse treatment program may be their only alternative to disciplinary action or dismissal (Trice & Beyer, 1984). When loss of productivity, rehabilitation costs, compensation costs, and extended negative social impact are considered in addition to morbidity figures, alcohol abuse is probably the major preventable expense of both business and government. Thus, increasing awareness of alcohol-related problems and encouraging early help-seeking behavior should have high priority in all organizations.

An encouraging aspect of EAPs is that their expanding focus and range of services has destigmatized an employee's seeking help for mental health and substance abuse problems. By including counseling for financial, legal, and family problems, EAPs are playing an increasingly important role in health promotion and mental wellness. Furthermore, many EAPs have broadened their initial emphasis on education and training to include aspects of health promotion other than substance abuse, thereby gaining added benefits of health promotion for their employees and their companies.

Increased Physical Activity

Cumulative evidence supports the efficacy of physical activity in reducing coronary heart disease and obesity as well as promoting physical function and mental well-being (Biddle, 1989). Heart disease, hypertension, and obesity are among the health concerns that have received the most attention. Many studies demonstrate that aerobic exercise leads to increased cardiac efficiency and reduced cardiovascular risk profiles (Kannel & Sorlie, 1979). Findings indicate that exercise can reduce cardiovascular risk factors including hypertension, high serum triglyceride levels, and high serum cholesterol levels (Paffenbarger & Hyde, 1984).

There is also evidence that exercise has beneficial effects on psychological functioning. Benefits associated with exercise most frequently include increased general well-being, reduced anxiety, depression, and muscle tension and improved mood, temperament, self-concept, and emotional stress tolerance (Blair, Jacobs, & Powell, 1985; Sime, 1984). The relationship between exercise and anxiety and depression has been extensively studied. However, few well-controlled experimental studies document program effects that imply an association between exercise and improved psychological functioning. Some studies do suggest that exercise has benefits in the management of psychological problems including anxiety, depression, and job-related stress (Sime, 1984). In addition, exercise has been shown to improve self-esteem, sense of control, cognitive functioning, and general moods (Sachs & Buffone, 1984) and may reduce symptoms of mild to moderate depression and anxiety and improve some Type A behaviors that lead to heart attacks (Taylor, Sallis, & Needle,1985).

Exercise has been utilized for both rehabilitative and preventive purposes. Some evidence indicates that direct but usually delayed physiological benefits are derived from exercise if it is conducted in sufficient duration, frequency, and intensity (Paffenbarger & Hyde, 1984), particularly in the prevention of cardiovascular heart disease (Gebhardt & Crump, 1990). A study by Blair, Piserchia, Wilbur, & Crowder (1986) reported that improvements in exercise and physical fitness were associated with beneficial changes in coronary heart disease risk factors, as well as in several psychosocial variables. The rehabilitative effects of exercise have been documented in individuals who have suffered from previous myocardial infarctions, hypertension, chronic obstructive lung disease, obesity, and diabetes (O'Donnell & Ainsworth, 1984). In a prospective study of back injuries in firemen, it was determined that individuals who scored highest in physical fitness had a significantly reduced incidence of back injuries than those who scored lowest (Cady, Thomas, & Karwasky, 1985).

There is extensive epidemiological evidence that physically active individuals are more successful at weight loss than those who are not physically active. Furthermore, exercise regimens produce a reliable and measurable effect on weight loss. They help prevent dietary relapse and maintain weight loss (Marlatt & Gordon, 1985).

Fitness Programs. Employer-sponsored exercise programs have proliferated in the past decade. Programs range in complexity from the distribution of exercise-related materials, brown-bag lectures, and employee-led exercise classes to comprehensive programs that include health screening, individual counseling, and complete exercise facilities. Though programs may involve both aerobic and nonaerobic exercise, aerobic exercise programs have received the most attention.

Employers are interested in the potential of exercise programs to reduce health care costs, absenteeism, and turnover and to increase employee productivity and improve corporate image. Benefits most commonly associated with participation in a regular exercise program are improvements in energy level, attitude toward job and employer, and self-rated work performance (Fielding, 1984). More recent research using control groups suggests a relationship between reductions in health care costs, absenteeism, and turnover and the implementation of comprehensive worksite programs that include physical activity (Gebhardt & Crump, 1990).

In a Canadian workplace, absenteeism was reduced by 22% and turnover by 14% when compared to a reference company (Cox, Shepard, & Corey, 1981). A study in Texas evaluating the impact of an exercise program for teachers reported 1.25 days less absenteeism for participants than for a comparison group (Blair et al., 1985). Other companies have also reported reduced absenteeism and turnover and improved attitude toward coworkers and supervisors (Keifhaber & Goldbeck, 1984; Lynch, Golaszewski, Clearie, Snow, & Vickery, 1990; Tsai, Bernacki, & Baun, 1988).

Though some studies have reported reduced absenteeism, most studies in this area have not had the scientific rigor necessary to establish unambiguously the specificity and overall effectiveness of exercise programs (O'Donnell & Ainsworth, 1984). Two serious limitations have been a strong self-selection bias and the lack of true control groups. A more recent study that examined the relationship between participation in a fitness program and absences found that program participants had a history of fewer absences before participation. At follow-up it was found that decrease in absenteeism depended on how many absences a participant had to begin with *and* how fully the individual participated in the fitness program (Lynch et al., 1990).

There is some evidence that exercise programs can benefit employees, but the cost benefit to employers is still debated (Blair et al., 1986; Mullen, Velez, Mains, Laville, & Biddle, 1989). There are positive changes in employee knowledge, behavior, attitudes, and physical measurements, but studies have not related these changes to employer cost savings (Kiefhaber & Goldbeck, 1984; Mullen et al., 1989). Most evaluation studies have utilized pre-experimental designs, which, by definition, do not provide the degree of scientific rigor necessary to establish the efficacy of an intervention. Thus, though there is evidence of individual psychological and physiological benefits to be gained from exercise, research has been inconclusive regarding the cost benefits to employers.

Merging Health Promotion Programs With Employee Benefits

Though there has been limited empirical evidence regarding the long-term benefits of most programs, promising short-term impacts have been noted. Continued support for worksite health promotion programs will depend on more effective implementation, better evaluation, and the incorporation of health promotion concepts and practices into the administrative philosophy and structure of companies.

Federal, state, and local public health agencies, as well as business coalitions and private foundations, have expended considerable effort to encourage businesses to adopt worksite disease prevention and health promotion programs (Berry, 1981; Kizer, 1987; National Chamber Foundation, 1978; O'Donnell & Ainsworth, 1984; Parkinson et al., 1982; Pelletier, Klehr, & McPhee, 1988; USDHHS, 1979b). Most of the early programs—those initiated in the 1960s—were offered on a one-shot basis which precluded the likelihood of any long-term effects (Nickerson, 1967). Another problem has been that many programs were initiated by outside agencies, such as commercial vendors and academic researchers, with only minimal company interest or involvement (Ware, 1982).

A number of exemplary comprehensive programs have been developed by large corporations including DuPont (Bertera, 1990), Johnson & Johnson (Blair et al., 1986; Jones, Bly, & Richardson, 1990; see chapter 11), General Mills (Wood, Olmstead, & Craig, 1989), and Tenneco (Tsai et al., 1988). These programs coordinate components such as smoking cessation, physical activity, and stress reduction into a coherent ongoing program. Data from these comprehensive interventions provide clear evidence that worksite programs reduce health risks and are cost effective (Pelletier, 1991).

Several factors affect the adoption and maintenance of health promotion programs in business and industry. These include the size of the organization, management perspective, priorities of the health care system, the structure of health insurance, and the position of organized labor.

Size of the Organization

Strongly associated with the offering of health promotion programs at worksites is the size of the company (USDHHS, 1987). Most of the elaborate programs cited in the literature as exemplary cases have been those of large corporations (Berry, 1981; Kiefhaber et al., 1979; O'Donnell & Ainsworth, 1984; Parkinson et al., 1982). National and regional surveys provide additional evidence of the relationship between size of company and availability of programs (Davis et al., 1984; Fielding & Breslow, 1983).

It is logical to assume that small businesses also would benefit from health promotion programs. Because most research and demonstration projects have been implemented in large companies, the findings seldom address the special needs and constraints of small companies. Given the dispersion and large number of persons employed in small businesses, the development of innovative health promotion programs needs to be stimulated in this sector, and the methods and outcomes associated with such programs actively disseminated (Yenny, 1984).

Management Perspective

Active support of top and middle management has been critical in the initiation of nearly all existing worksite health promotion programs. A major stimulus for management's increased involvement in health has been the rapid rise of costs for medical services. Health promotion programs represent a potential strategy to help reduce health care costs.

Executives also see other potential benefits of health promotion programs. These include improved image of the organization, as seen both by employees and by those outside the company, reduction of human resource development costs by gaining an edge in recruitment and retention of employees, and improved employee morale and productivity. Program adoption often has been based at first on the potential of the programs to contribute to a better company image. Thus, image-conscious companies have adopted health promotion policies most readily. Related to image but as an additional impetus, the type of products or services that a company offers the public sometimes influences its employee programs. It is clearly in the interest of a company that produces athletic equipment to encourage exercise and fitness among its employees and to maintain a high profile in this area.

Several general factors pose constraints to program development. For example, the financial status of a company strongly influences its willingness and ability to initiate programs. A firm that is in the black may be more willing to incur new expenses without guarantee of recovery of costs than would be one that is running in the red. Other companies are unwilling to invest money in programs without strong, concrete evidence of economic benefits. Then, too, many decision-makers hesitate to propose anything that does not fit into existing administrative and budgetary procedures.

There still is considerable skepticism about the appropriateness of providing certain health education and health promotion programs at worksites. Some executives and managers feel that programs would be perceived negatively by employees and unions as infringements on rights. There are concerns about liability for accidents and injuries to employees while participating in programs, especially exercise and fitness programs. In some cases, individuals and unions strongly resist the collection of what they consider "confidential" information, such as personal smoking habits and alcohol and other drug use. Related to this issue is the frequent difficulty in gaining access to attendance records and insurance claims records. Inability or difficulty in collecting good baseline data makes it hard to set goals and priorities and to evaluate programs.

Sometimes employers fear that extra screening of employees may identify health problems that are related to the workplace, which again raises liability issues. Finally, there is the problem of conflicts of interest. Producers of products that are established health risks, such as cigarettes, must weigh the promotion of their product against the protection of the health of their employees and their families. Unfortunately, cigarette producers often either directly encourage smoking by providing free or discounted cigarettes or indirectly by not restricting smoking in the workplace or by not offering smoking cessation programs.

The likelihood that any program will be provided is based on management consideration of a fairly complex array of positive and negative factors. Selection of particular programs and the relative emphasis placed on them often depends on factors other than accurate assessments of employee needs. Given the difficulty of demonstrating cost benefits, especially in small businesses, the situation is not likely to change unless outside subsidies or incentives are provided. This presents a great challenge for both public and private sector organizations involved in preventive medicine and health promotion.

The Health Care System

The traditional role of physicians, and the major focus of most modern medical training, is the diagnosis and treatment of disease and the care of the individual patient. Thus, most physicians have little training in preventive medicine or public health. The result is that many medical departments in large organizations have been run like medical clinics rather than preventive or public health services.

Within the last 10 years, physicians and hospitals have shown signs of accepting health promotion as a legitimate component of medicine and even as a potentially lucrative extension of medical or hospital practice. Medical and hospital receptivity have much to do with the credibility of health promotion within the health care system (Cataldo et al., 1986; Green, Wilson, & Lovato, 1986). With the growing interest and support of these groups, worksite health promotion has a viable future.

Though there are political and financial reasons for physicians to maintain a strong clinical and treatment bias, there is also frequent criticism of this strategy in company-based medical departments. The more active involvement in medical and health care issues of business leaders in dialogue with a variety of nonmedical consultants has begun to counterbalance the once exclusive influence of organized medicine on health policy decisions. As a result, management mandates for a more preventive philosophy and expansion of preventive services is fostering the development by existing medical departments of more health education and health promotion programming.

Cost Containment.   When the cost of health care passed a critical threshold in the late 1970s, economists and major business leaders suddenly became more concerned with the structure of health care benefit plans and the utilization of services. Escalating costs have spawned widespread implementation of a variety of cost-containment strategies, one of which is corporate health promotion.

Strategies such as cost-shifting and cost-sharing have become very popular cost-containment methods. Many employers are raising the deductibles and copayment on health insurance plans and are requiring that employees get second and third opinions before undergoing surgery. Employees not only are being educated to become more frugal consumers of health care, but also are being discouraged from using some services. This strategy can provide short-term benefits but may be detrimental when deferred costs are considered.

Given the nature of today's major health problems and the structure of the medical care system, there is a limit to the savings that can be realized through these cost-containment measures. The current enthusiasm for short-term, moderate cost-containment strategies is drawing some attention and funds away from disease prevention and health promotion programs. Thus, control of rising costs through expedient financial methods has become the primary strategy of the employee benefits planners of most organizations. This, however, may be only a temporary palliative.

Health Insurance Incentives.   Early health insurance programs were designed to cover a portion of hospital costs, which generally were the most expensive part of medical care. The goal of these programs was to guarantee medical care to persons who were able to pay premiums on a continuing basis. Group plans covering all the employees of participating companies reduced average premiums and extended coverage to most American workers. This was viewed by some as the dawning of a new era of health for the rank and file.

Most insurance plans have restricted the options of the insured to select medical services. Plans with an exclusive emphasis on cure really are not health plans, they are sickness-cost insurance intended to prepay the cost of medical care. They offer little that would help keep healthy people well and, hence, out of hospital beds. Even simple diagnostic and therapeutic procedures that could be managed easily in a general practice office are carried out in the hospital if the patient happens to be covered by hospitalization. Thus, medical costs have continued to climb.

Over the last 20 years, employee benefit plans were progressively changed to give employees broader benefits. These plans primarily cover expensive, high-technology diagnosis and treatment of disease—not its prevention. Typical benefit plans pay 100% for emergency room costs, 80% or less for inpatient and outpatient care, and usually nothing for preventive health services. Because health promotion activities are neither adverse nor unpredicted, they fall outside the current concept of insurance (Hosokawa, 1984).

The increasing evidence for the effectiveness and, in some cases, cost benefit of selected health promotion services has had little impact on benefit planning. In most cases, the health promotion programs and services provided by companies have not been covered by prepaid health insurance benefits (Kiefhaber et al., 1979). Such programs and services, therefore, represent new costs to employers unless provided free or at nominal cost by outside agencies or if employees themselves pay for the programs.

It is generally assumed that insurance coverage for health promotion services and programs is highly desirable. The advisability of this, however, is questionable (Kiefhaber & Goldbeck, 1984). It may be counterproductive to seek insurance coverage for health promotion programs at present because of a proposed tax cap on the amount of employee benefits for health insurance. Currently, these programs are outside the cap, because they are an uninsured benefit. Kiefhaber and Goldbeck (1984) argue that if these programs were inside the cap, they would probably be among the first programs to be eliminated by many large companies, because, as they do not represent immediate health needs, they could be more ethically and conveniently reduced than could medical or surgical services.

Another issue related to insurance is that of using adjustments in insurance premiums as a means of motivating employees to participate in health programs and to make changes in their health habits. This is a complex issue, which has both positive and negative aspects. On the plus side, financial incentives, if sufficiently large, often motivate persons to make changes that they otherwise would not make. Incentives for nonsmokers are already being written into many insurance plans, but they are relatively low, and there is no evidence that they decrease smoking. On the minus side, actuarial predictions based on large samples are reliable, but individual risk estimation is inaccurate. Thus, individuals could and should challenge any uprating of their premiums. Penalizing individuals for health risk behaviors also invites negative responses from labor.

Labor Perspective

The perspective of organized labor must be considered when assessing the future of worksite-based health promotion programs. Most statements and articles on health promotion represent the programmatic views of either government or management. Organized labor has not had a high profile in health promotion, but it is in a strong position to either foster or hamper the development of programs.

In the past, organized labor has been influential in bringing about many improvements in work conditions related to safety and health. Both management and labor have an interest in the health and welfare of the work force, but often their views on how best to accomplish this have differed. This appears to be the case with current health promotion programs.

One of the greatest concerns expressed by labor groups has been the question of "blaming the victim," particularly for those workers who are exposed to potentially health-threatening conditions, such as the presence of harmful chemicals in the workplace. The concern here is that employers will use the concepts of behavior change and worker responsibility for health as smoke screens to cover neglect of hazards in the work environment. Efforts directed at teaching risk-reducing practices and behaviors to workers, combined with managerial policy and environmental reforms to improve working conditions, are the most desirable approach.

An advantage of a combined educational and environmental approach is that some worksite hazards interact with worker behavior. Some are synergistic in their effects, such as smoking and exposure to asbestos, solvents, and other air pollutants. Some have corollary effects on health problems, such as alcohol use and risk of injury. Some may affect worker productivity and health similarly but independently, as do stressful working conditions, being overweight, or being sedentary and lacking physical fitness. These interactions between working conditions and health behavior call for a comprehensive approach to worksite health promotion that will provide interventions directed at protecting the worker against hazardous and stressful working conditions and promoting healthful practices, such as exercise, proper diet, and self-examination for cancer signs or symptoms (Sloan, Gruman, & Allegrante, 1987).

Summary

Health promotion in the corporate environment can be justified from a public health perspective, but the acceptance of programs by corporations depends on more than epidemiological evidence and evaluative research. A hierarchy of priorities, including account costs and benefits accruing to the firm, as well as public relations considerations and employee needs and enthusiasm, must be satisfied.

Major factors influencing the caution with which many organizations have advocated health promotion programs include questions about the relative importance of the many problems being targeted and serious doubts about the effectiveness and quality of the programs being offered. Health promotion programs have become highly commercialized, producing a great deal of competition among providers and vendors. There is good reason for potential purchasers to beware the admonition, caveat emptor.

The challenge now facing both management and labor is to reduce the incidence and prevalence of many of the most common causes of medical care by establishing comprehensive, long-term disease prevention and health promotion programs. To be successful, a health promotion program must be integrated with the overall benefit planning strategy of an organization or union. The objectives should be reasonable and attainable, within reach of a company's financial resources, and aligned with its overall philosophy and goals.

Prospects for the proliferation of such programs are bright. They are popular with employees, and they supply management with positive, constructive, relatively low-cost benefits for employees. Also, they improve both health and productivity indicators in the short term and may reduce medical care expenditures in the long term. The prospects for effective change depend in part on the strengthening of scientific evidence of the effectiveness of health promotion strategies and in part on the training of personnel to implement these strategies effectively in the workplace.

Note

Portions of this chapter were presented at the Harvard Symposium on Health Promotion in the Workplace, Boston, October 8-10, 1986. Preparation of this paper was supported in part by NIH grant T32-HLO7555-03 and by the National Institute for Occupational Safety and Health. The authors were with the Center for Health Promotion Research and Development at the University of Texas Health Science Center at Houston when the original version of this chapter was written.

References

Aguirre-Molina, M., & Molina, C. (1990). Ethnic/racial populations and worksite health promotion. *Occupational Medicine, 5,* 789-805.

American Lung Association. (1982). *Occupational health legislation and regulation: A progress report* (ALA Memo-34). New York: Author.

Ardell, D. (1979). *High level wellness: An alternative to doctors, drugs, and disease.* New York: Bantam Books.

Ardell, D. (1984). The history and future of wellness. *Wellness Perspectives,* **1**, 3-23.

Backer, T. (1987). *Strategic planning for workplace drug abuse programs* (DHHS Publication No. ADM 87-1538). Rockville, MD: National Institute on Drug Abuse.

Bennett, D., & Levy, B. (1980). Smoking policies and smoking cessation programs of large employers in Massachusetts. *American Journal of Public Health,* **70**, 629-631.

Berry, C. (1981). *Good health for employers and reduced health care costs for industry.* Washington, DC: Health Insurance Association of America.

Bertera, R. (1990). The effects of workplace health promotion on absenteeism and employee costs in a large industrial population. *American Journal of Public Health,* **80**, 1101-1105.

Bertera, R., Oehl, L., & Telepchak, J. (1990). Self-help versus group approaches to smoking cessation in the workplace: Eighteen-month follow-up and cost analysis. *American Journal of Health Promotion,* **4**,187-192.

Bibeau, D., Mullen K., McLeroy, K., Green, L., & Foshee, V. (1988). Evaluations of workplace smoking cessation programs: A critique. *American Journal of Preventive Medicine,* **4**, 87-95.

Biddle, S., & Fox, K. (1989). Exercise and health psychology: Emerging relationships. *British Journal of Medical Psychology,* **62**(3), 205-216.

Blair, S., Jacobs, D., Jr., & Powell, K. (1985). Relationships between exercise or physical activity and other health behaviors. *Public Health Reports,* **100**, 172-180.

Blair, S., Piserchia, P., Wilbur, C., & Crowder, J. (1986). A public health intervention model for work-site health promotion: Impact on exercise and physical fitness in a health promotion plan after 24 months. *Journal of the American Medical Association,* **255**, 921-926.

Brody, B. (1988). Employee assistance programs: An historical and literature review. *American Journal of Health Promotion,* **2**(3), 13-19.

Bunker, J., Eriksen, M., & Kinsey, J. (1987, September). AIDS in the workplace: The role of EAP's. *The Almacan,* pp. 18-26.

Cady, L., Thomas, P., & Karwasky, R. (1985). Program for increasing health and physical fitness of fire fighters. *Journal of Occupational Medicine,* **27**, 110-114.

Caplan, G., & Killilea, M. (Eds.) (1976). *Support systems and mutual help: Multidisciplinary explorations.* New York: Grune & Stratton.

Carey, K., & Abrams, D. (1988). Properties of saliva cotinine in light smokers. *American Journal of Public Health,* **78**, 842-843.

Cataldo, M., Green, L., Herd, J., Parkinson, R., & Goldbeck, W. (1986). Preventive medicine and the corporate environment: Challenge to behavioral medicine. In M. Cataldo & T. Coates (Eds.), *Health and industry: A behavioral medicine perspective* (pp. 399-419). New York: Wiley.

Cook, R., & Youngblood, A. (1990). Preventing substance abuse as an integral part of worksite health promotion. *Occupational Medicine, 5,* 725-738.

Cox, M., Shepard, R., & Corey, P. (1981). Influence of an employee fitness program upon fitness, productivity, and absenteeism. *Ergonomics, 24,* 795-806.

Cunningham, R. (1982). *Wellness at work.* Chicago: Blue Cross Association.

Danaher, B. (1982). Smoking cessation programs in occupational settings. In R. Parkinson & Associates (Eds.), *Managing health promotion in the workplace.* Palo Alto, CA: Mayfield.

Davis, M., Rosenberg, K., Iverson, D., Vernon, T., & Bauer, J. (1984). Worksite health promotion in Colorado. *Public Health Reports, 99,* 538-543.

Dubos, R. (1959). *Mirage of health: Utopias, progress and biological change.* New York: Harper & Row.

Dunkin, W. (1982). *The employee assistance manual.* New York: National Council on Alcoholism.

Dupont, R., & Basen, M. (1982). Control of alcohol and drug abuse. In R. Parkinson & Associates (Eds.), *Managing health promotion in the workplace* (pp. 194-232). Palo Alto, CA: Mayfield.

Eriksen, M. (1986). Workplace smoking control: Rationale and approaches. In W. Ward (Ed.), *Advances in health education and promotion* (pp. 65-103). Greenwich, CO: JAI Press.

Eriksen, M., LeMaistre, C., & Newell, G. (1988). Health hazards of passive smoking. *Annual Review of Public Health, 9,* 47-70.

Fielding, J. (1984). Health promotion and disease prevention at the worksite. *Annual Review of Public Health, 5,* 237-265.

Fielding, J. (1990). Worksite health promotion survey: Smoking control activities. *Preventive Medicine, 19,* 402-413.

Fielding, J. (1991). Smoking control at the workplace. *Annual Review of Public Health, 12,* 209-234.

Fielding, J., & Breslow, L. (1983). Health promotion programs sponsored by California employers. *American Journal of Public Health, 73,* 538-542.

Fielding, J., & Piserchia, P. (1989). Frequency of worksite health promotion activities. *American Journal of Public Health, 79,* 16-20.

Gebhardt, D., & Crump, C. (1990). Employee fitness and wellness programs in the workplace. *American Psychologist, 45*(2), 262-272.

Giesbrecht, N., Gonzales, R., Grant, M., Osterberg, E., Room, R., Rootman, I., & Towle, L. (Eds.) (1988). *Drinking and casualties: Accidents, poisoning and violence in an international perspective.* London: Droom Helm.

Gottlieb, N., Eriksen, M., Lovato, C., Weinstein, R., & Green, L. (1990). Impact of a restrictive worksite smoking policy on smoking behavior, attitudes, and norms. *Journal of Occupational Medicine*, **32**(1), 16-23.

Green, L. (1980). Healthy people: The Surgeon General's report and the prospects. In W. McNerney (Ed.), *Working for a healthier America* (pp. 95-110). Cambridge, MA: Ballinger.

Green, L., Wilson, A., & Lovato, C. (1986). What changes can health promotion achieve and how long do these changes last? The trade-offs between expediency and durability. *Preventive Medicine*, **15**, 508-521.

Hosokawa, M. (1984). Insurance incentives for health promotion. *Health Education*, **15**, 9-12.

Illich, I. (1976). *Medical nemesis*. New York: Pantheon.

Jones, R., Bly, J., & Richardson, J. (1990). A study of worksite health promotion programs and absenteeism. *Journal of Occupational Medicine*, **32**, 95-99.

Kannel, W., & Sorlie, P. (1979). Some health benefits of physical activity. The Framingham Study. *Archives of Internal Medicine*, **139**, 857-861.

Kiefhaber, A., & Goldbeck, W. (1984). *Worksite wellness. Prospects for a healthier America*. Washington, DC: U.S. Department of Health & Human Services.

Kiefhaber, A., Weinberg, A., & Goldbeck, W. (1979). *A survey of industry sponsored health promotion, prevention, and education programs*. Washington, DC: Washington Business Group for Health.

Kizer, W. (1987). *The healthy workplace: A blueprint for corporate action*. New York: Wiley.

Klarreich, S., Francek, J., & Moore, C. (Eds.) (1985). *The human resources management handbook: Principles and practices of employer assistance programs*. New York: Praeger.

Knowles, J. (Ed.) (1977). *Doing better and feeling worse: Health in the U.S.* New York: Norton.

Kotz, H., & Fielding, J. (Eds.) (1980). *Health, education, and promotion: Agenda for the eighties*. Summary report of an insurance industry conference on health education and promotion (sponsored by the Health Insurance Association of America), Atlanta, Georgia, March 16-18.

Kristein, M. (1983). How much can business expect to profit from smoking cessation? *Preventive Medicine*, **12**, 358-381.

Kurtz, N., Googins, B., & Howard, H. (1984). Measuring the success of occupational alcoholism programs. *Journal of Studies on Alcohol*, **45**, 33-45.

Laframboise, H. (1973). Health policy: Breaking it down into more manageable segments. *Canadian Medical Association Journal*, **108**, 388-393.

Lalonde, M. (1974). *A new perspective on the health of Canadians* (Cat. No. H31-1374). Ottawa: Ministry of Health and Welfare.

Levin, L., Katz, A., & Holst, E. (1976). *Self-care: Lay initiatives in health.* New York: Prodist.

Lynch, W., Golaszewski, T., Clearie, A., Snow, D., & Vickery, D. (1990). Impact of a facility-based corporate fitness program on the number of absences from work due to illness. *Journal of Occupational Medicine,* **32**(1), 9-12.

Marlatt, G., & Gordon, J. (1985). *Relapse prevention.* New York: Guilford Press.

McGinnis, J. (1982). Targeting progress in health. *Public Health Reports,* **97**, 295.

McKeown, T. (1971). *A historical appraisal of the medical task. Medical history and medical care.* New York: Oxford University Press.

McLeroy, K., Green, L., Mullen, K., & Foshee, V. (1984). Assessing the effects of health promotion in worksites: A review of stress program evaluations. *Health Education Quarterly,* **11**, 379-401.

McNerney, W. (Ed.) (1980). *Working for a healthier America.* Cambridge, MA: Ballinger.

Mullen, P., Velez, R., Mains, D., Laville, E., & Biddle, A. (1989). *Meta-analysis of patient education for cardiovascular disease patients.* (Report). San Antonio: Audie L. Murphy Memorial Veterans Administration Hospital.

Naditch, M. (1984). The StayWell Program. In J. Matarazzo, S. Weiss, A. Herd, & N. Miller (Eds.), *Behavioral health: A handbook of health enhancement and disease prevention* (pp. 1071-1078). New York: Wiley.

National Institute on Alcohol Abuse and Alcoholism. (1984). *Fifth special report to the U.S. Congress on alcohol and health* (DHHS Publication No. ADM 84-1291). Washington, DC: U.S. Government Printing Office.

Nickerson, H. (1967). An evaluation of health education programs in occupational settings. *Health Education Monograph,* **22**, 16-31.

O'Donnell, M., & Ainsworth, T. (Eds.) (1984). *Health promotion in the workplace.* New York: Wiley.

Orleans, C., & Shipley, R. (1982). Worksite smoking initiatives: Review and recommendations. *Addictive Behaviors,* **7**, 1-16.

Paffenbarger, R., Jr., & Hyde, R. (1984). Exercise in the prevention of coronary heart disease. *Preventive Medicine,* **13**, 3-22.

Parkinson, R., Green, L., McGill, A., Eriksen, M., Ware, B., & Associates (Eds.) (1982). *Managing health promotion in the workplace: Guidelines for implementation and evaluation.* Palo Alto, CA: Mayfield.

Pelletier, K. (1979). *Holistic medicine.* New York: Delta.

Pelletier, K. (1991). A review and analysis of the health and cost-effectiveness outcome studies of comprehensive health promotion and disease prevention programs. *American Journal of Health Promotion,* **5**, 311-313.

Pelletier, K., Klehr, N., & McPhee, S. (1988). Town and gown: A lesson in collaboration. *Business and Health,* **6**, 34-39.

Public Health Reports (1980). *Health promotion programs in occupational settings: A special section*, **95**, 96-163.

Roizen, J. (1982). *Estimating alcohol involvement in serious events. Alcohol consumption and alcohol problems* (DHHS Publication No. ADM 82-1190). Washington, DC: U.S. Government Printing Office.

Ross, C., Sherman, S., Ber, K., Radbill, L., Lee, E., Giloth, B., Jones, L., & Longe, M. (1985, August). Health promotion programs flourishing: Survey. *Hospital*, pp. 128-135.

Sachs, M., & Buffone, G. (Eds.) (1984). *Running as therapy*. Lincoln, NE: University of Nebraska Press.

Sehnert, K., & Tillotson, J. (1978). *How business can promote good health for employees and their families: A national health care strategy*. Washington, DC: National Chamber Foundation.

Shimp, D. (1978, July/August). Nonsmoker rights in the workplace: A new look. *American Lung Association Bulletin*, pp. 3-6.

Shipley R., Orleans, C., Wilbur, C., Piserchia, P., & McFadden D. (1988). Effect of the Johnson & Johnson LIVE FOR LIFE Program on employee smoking. *Preventive Medicine*, **17**, 25-34.

Sime, W. (1984). Psychological benefits of exercise training in the healthy individual. In J. Matarazzo, S. Weiss, J. Herd, & N. Miller (Eds.), *Behavioral health: A handbook of health enhancement and disease prevention*. New York: Wiley.

Sloan R., Gruman, J., & Allegrante, J. (1987). *Investing in employee health: A guide to effective health promotion in the workplace*. San Francisco: Jossey-Bass.

Spicer, J. (Ed.) (1987). *The EAP solution: Current trends and future solutions*. Center City, MN: Hazelden Foundation.

Taylor, C., Sallis, J., & Needle, R. (1985). The relation of physical activity and exercise to mental health. *Public Health Reports*, **100**, 195-202.

Trice, H., & Beyer, J. (1984). Work-related outcomes of the constructive-confrontation strategy in a job-based alcoholism program. *Journal of Studies on Alcohol*, **45**, 393-404.

Tsai, S., Bernacki, E., & Baun, W. (1988). Injury prevalence and associated costs among participants of an employee fitness program. *Preventive Medicine*, **17**, 475-482.

U.S. Department of Health and Human Services. (1978). *Report of the president's commission on mental health*. Washington, DC: U.S. Government Printing Office.

U.S. Department of Health and Human Services. (1979a). *Healthy people: The Surgeon General's report on health promotion and disease prevention* (DHEW PHS Publication No. 79-55071). Washington, DC: U.S. Government Printing Office.

U.S. Department of Health and Human Services. (1979b). *Proceedings of the national conference on health promotion programs in occupational settings* (SN Publication No. 630-389-2562). Washington, DC: U.S. Government Printing Office.

U.S. Department of Health and Human Services. (1980). *Promoting health/ preventing disease: Objectives for the nation* (Publication No. 1981 0-349-256). Washington, DC: U.S. Government Printing Office.

U.S. Department of Health and Human Services. (1984). *Prospects for a healthier America: Achieving the nation's health promotion objectives.* Washington, DC: U.S. Office of Disease Prevention and Health Promotion.

U.S. Department of Health and Human Services. (1986). *The health consequences of involuntary smoking: A report of the surgeon general.* (DHHS Publication No. PHS 87-8398). Washington, DC: U.S. Government Printing Office.

U.S. Department of Health and Human Services. (1987). *National survey of worksite health promotion activities: A summary.* Washington, DC: U.S. Government Printing Office.

U.S. Department of Health and Human Services. (1989a). *Reducing the health consequences of smoking: 25 years of progress. A report of the Surgeon General* (DHHS Publication No. PHS 89-8411). Washington, DC: U.S. Government Printing Office.

U.S. Department of Health and Human Services. (1989b). *U.S. Surgeon General's workshop on drunk driving: Background papers.* Washington, DC: U.S. Government Printing Office.

U.S. Department of Health and Human Services. (1991). *Healthy people 2000: National health promotion and disease prevention objectives* (DHHS Publication No. PHS 91-50212). Washington, DC: U.S. Government Printing Office.

U.S. Department of Labor. (1992). New BLS projections: Findings and implications. In *Outlook: 1990-2005.* Bureau of Labor Statistics. Bulletin 2402, May, 1992.

Vojtecky, M., Kar, S., & Cox, S. (1985). Workplace health education: Results from a national survey. *International Journal of Community Health Education, 5,* 171-185.

Walsh, D., & Gordon, N. (1986). Legal approaches to smoking deterrence. *Annual Review of Public Health, 7,* 127-149.

Walsh, D., & Kelleher, S. (1987). *Preventing alcohol and drug abuse through programs at the workplace.* Washington, DC: Washington Business Group on Health.

Ware, B. (1982). Health education in occupational settings: History has a message. *Health Education Quarterly* (special supplement), *9,* 37-41.

Warner, K. (1987). Health and economic implications of a tobacco-free society. *Journal of the American Medical Association, 258*(15), 2080-2086.

Warner, K., & Murt, H. (1984). Economic incentives for health. *Annual Review of Public Health, 5,* 107-133.

Weisbrod, R.R., Pirie, P.L., Bracht, N.F., & Elstun, P. (1991). Worksite health promotion in four Midwest cities. *Journal of Community Health*, **16**(3), 169-77.

Windsor, R., & Bartlett, E. (1984). Employee self-help smoking cessation programs: A review of the literature. *Health Education Quarterly*, **11**, 349-359.

Wood, E., Olmstead, G., & Craig, J. (1989). An evaluation of lifestyle risk factors and absenteeism after two years in a worksite health promotion program. *American Journal of Health Promotion*, **4**(2), 128-133.

Yenny, S. (1984). *Small businesses and health promotion*. New York: National Center for Health Education.

Yenny, S., & Behrens, R. (1984). *Health promotion and business coalitions: Current activities and prospects for the future*. Washington, DC: U.S. Department of Health and Human Services.

Chapter 2

Positioning Health Promotion to Make an Economic Impact

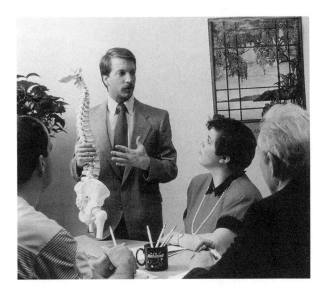

David Chenoweth

What is the future of American business? A day rarely passes that we don't hear of another layoff, labor strike, corporate takeover, bankruptcy, or plant closing. The issue of rising health care costs is closely related to many of these events and appears to be a top concern for both employees and employers as both groups are picking up higher percentages of the nation's health care bill. For example, American employers pay approximately 40% of the tab compared to 18% in 1965. The result is that nearly half of all business profits are spent on health care services (see Figure 2.1).

Although health care cost inflation has slowed since 1984—climbing at an annual rate of almost 9%—health care cost increases continue to rise two to three times faster than general inflation. Moreover, health care

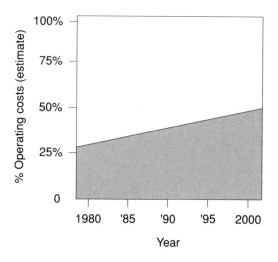

Figure 2.1   Business spending for health care services as a percentage of corporate operating profits. *Note.* Data from Health Care Financing Administration and Department of Commerce. Estimate provided by Health Management Associates.

spending will climb to about 1-1/2 trillion dollars by the year 2000 and take up 18%—or more, according to some analysts—of the nation's gross domestic product (see Figure 2.2).

As health care cost-control efforts intensify in the 1990s, employers will face tough decisions on how to control these costs without compromising benefits and employee morale. In creating an offensive strategy, senior management must realize that health care costs are driven primarily by strong economic forces that are not easily influenced by corporate policies and employees' actions.

- Inflation is a major driving force. The medical care services component of the consumer price index (CPI) continues to rise two to three times faster than does the index as a whole (see Figure 2.3). In fact, some economists estimate that medical care inflation alone accounts for as much as one third of rising health care costs.
- Cost-shifting accounts for nearly 30% of increased costs. Hospitals and doctors pass along the costs of unpaid bills, under the guise of price increases, to patients who have health insurance coverage and thus to their employers (Business & Health, 1990).
- Greater utilization of medical care services accounts for about 16% of increased costs. As more Americans live longer and use more health care services in their later years, this figure, too, will rise (Business & Health, 1990).

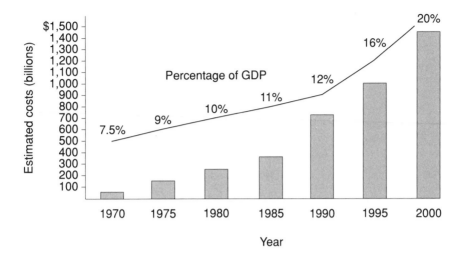

Figure 2.2 United States health care expenditures and their percentage of the gross domestic product. *Note.* Data from Health Care Financing Administration. Estimates for 1992-1996 provided by the Department of Commerce and for 1997-2000 by Health Management Associates.

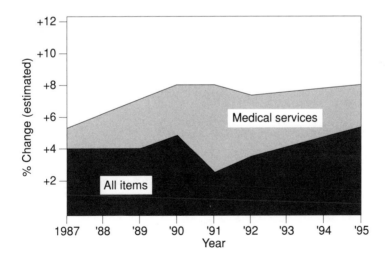

Figure 2.3 Annual percentage changes in the medical care services component of the consumer price index compared to all items in the index. *Note.* Data from Bureau of Labor Statistics and Department of Commerce. Estimates by Health Management Associates.

- New technology is another factor (e.g., CAT scanning, MRI, and lasers) that inflates health care cost another 12% (Business & Health, 1990).
- Catastrophic cases such as transplant operations, AIDS, kidney dialysis, and care of premature infants boost health care costs approximately 9% (Business & Health, 1990).
- Medical malpractice insurance premiums and use of "defensive" medicine are estimated to inflate health care costs another 1% to 2% (Business & Health, 1990).

Because today's health care costs are driven primarily by strong economic forces, health promotion activities must be integrated with other cost-control strategies, such as hospitalization control, managed care, cost-sharing, and consumer education, if they are to help keep future health care costs within bounds.

Integrating Health Management

For many organizations, the most efficient and cost-effective approach is to include health promotion activities in an integrated health management framework (see Figure 2.4). In fact, some of America's best-known companies, such as Adolph Coors, Kimberly-Clark, Quaker Oats, Northern Telecom, and Southern California Edison, operate health management frameworks to enhance their health promotion and cost-control efforts.

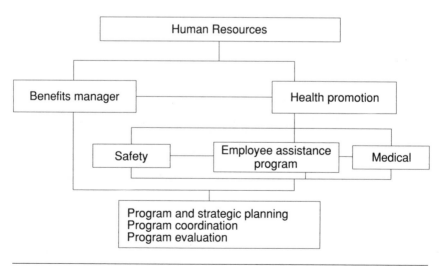

Figure 2.4 A sample health management framework in a midsized company.

Integrated health management frameworks essentially offer organizations greater cost-control potential than nonintegrated frameworks (see Figure 2.5). For example, from 1985 to 1990, I studied the impact of integrated health management frameworks in seven large companies and found that health care costs increased an average of 7.5% per year—just one third the national average (see Figure 2.6). These cost savings gave each company more money to invest in research and development, employee training, and pay increases (Chenoweth, 1991a).

The following profiles illustrate the various health promotion and cost-control components that constitute actual health management frameworks used in three organizations—a small business, a midsized company, and a large industry.

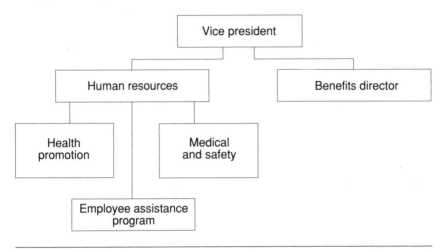

Figure 2.5   An example of a nonintegrated health management approach in a midsized company.

Profile of a Small Company—
The Robert E. Mason Company

The Robert E. Mason Company is a Charlotte, North Carolina–based company with 75 employees. Two employees, the operations manager and the sales secretary, are given release time to administer the company's health promotion programs (see Table 2.1). The company president has final approval over programs and expenditures. The operations manager serves as a member of the human resources team as well as the quality implementation team. Both teams could eventually be involved in program decisions, but to date, these groups offer support only. Figure 2.7 shows this company's health management framework.

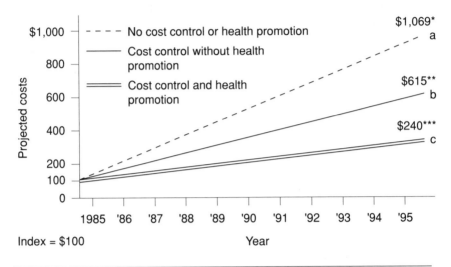

Figure 2.6 What $100 of health care services cost from 1985 to 1995 in companies with (a) no cost-control or health promotion programs, (b) cost-control programs without health promotion, and (c) cost-control and health promotion programs. *Note.* From David H. Chenoweth, PhD, *Planning Health Promotion at the Worksite*, 2d ed. Copyright © Wm. C. Brown Communications, Inc., Dubuque, Iowa. All Rights Reserved. Reprinted by permission. *Based on the average annual health care cost increase of 20% for American employers during 1985-1990. **Based on an annual health care cost increase of 15% on the assumption that cost-control measures have slowed annual cost increases from 20% to 15%. ***Based on the average annual health care cost increase of 7.5% from 1983 to 1990 of seven companies (Adolph Coors, Caterpillar, Kimberly-Clark, Lord Corporation, Mesa Petroleum, Southern California Edison, and The Quaker Oats Company).

Table 2.1
Health Management Personnel and Key Responsibilities
of Robert E. Mason Company

Personnel	Primary duties	% of workload
Operations manager	Health promotion program	10
	Human resources, personnel, and health insurance administration	90
Sales secretary	Aerobic instructor	10
	Administrative sales	90

Note. Data from Robert E. Mason Company, Charlotte, NC.

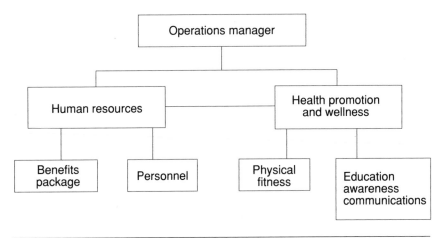

Figure 2.7   The health management framework used at the Robert E. Mason Company. *Note.* Data from Robert E. Mason Company, Charlotte, NC.

According to Elaine Coleman, the company's operations manager, "It is very difficult for us to measure the impact of health promotion on employees' health and overall cost management goals. In any event, we have more employees participating in the health fair each year, and more family members becoming involved with our program. Only in the last year have we been measuring 'sick days' of employees, so it will be a while before data is available for real measurement. We do know our preemployment physical and reimbursement for physicals detected cancer in its earliest stages in two of our people.

"In 1987, our insurance provider decreased a rate increase by 5% due to our health promotion program. They have been so pleased with our program that our premium rates have been directly tied to our claims experience; therefore, our increases have been minimized and not on a yearly basis as with many of their clients" (personal communication, 1991; see Figure 2.8). "We have had to increase the employee deductible over the past 3 years as well as the employee's out-of-pocket maximum. We try to encourage our employees to be good consumers of health care services, but this is very difficult."

Profile of a Medium-Sized Company— The Lord Corporation

Lord Corporation is headquartered in Erie, Pennsylvania with a work force of approximately 1,600 employees; about one fourth of Lord's employees work at the company's research and development facility in Cary,

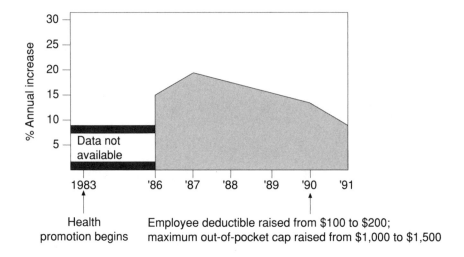

Figure 2.8   Annual health care cost increases for Robert E. Mason Company. *Note.* Data from Robert E. Mason Company, Charlotte, NC.

North Carolina, and at Lord's manufacturing plants in Dayton, Ohio, Shelton, Connecticut, and Bowling Green, Kentucky. See Figure 2.9 and Table 2.2 for the company's health management framework.

Ruth Shindledecker, manager of employee benefits at Lord states, "Our health and wellness programs have helped to make our employees more intelligent health care consumers, based on feedback from providers. Because we are self-insured, our health care costs vary widely from year to year with the effect of catastrophic cases" (see Figure 2.10).

"We began our cost-containment program in 1983 by reducing dental benefits, introducing managed care, [and initiating] an ongoing and extensive communication campaign and a gain-sharing incentive concept. In 1989 we changed to a new inpatient hospital administrator, limited inpatient psychiatric and chiropractic benefits, set dollar limits on our overall coverage, [and] secured union agreement for direct contracting and a 'defined dollar' retiree program tied to service. Various safety, wellness, and consumer education programs are ongoing. Overall, an integrated health management approach in which all staff members work together is the major reason for our cost-control success in the past decade" (personal communication, 1991).

Profile of a Large Industry— The Quaker Oats Company

The Quaker Oats Company is located in Chicago, Illinois, and has approximately 17,000 employees nationwide. (See Figure 2.11 and Table 2.3 for

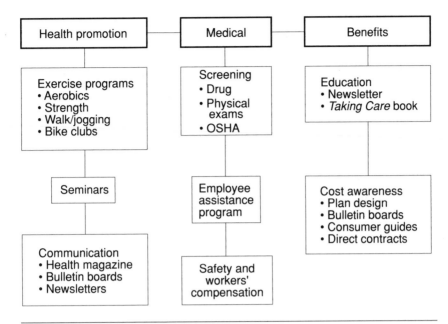

Figure 2.9 The health management framework at Lord Corporation. *Note.* Data from The Lord Corporation, Erie, PA.

Table 2.2
Health Management Personnel and Key Responsibilities
of the Lord Corporation

Personnel	Primary functions
Manager, Human Resource staff	Oversees health, wellness, benefits, and workers' compensation
Manager, Employee Benefits	Administers all benefit programs; coordinates health, wellness, and cost communications
Manager, Health Services	Coordinates nursing services, screening, physicals, drug and OSHA testing, EAP and workers' compensation
Employee Assistance Program	Contracts for counselors at various work locations
Employee Relations staff	Carries out decentralized approach to workers' compensation and safety

Note. Data from the Lord Corporation, Erie, PA.

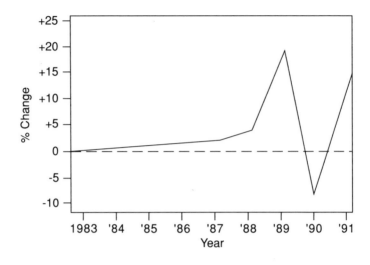

Figure 2.10   Annual health care cost increases at Lord Corporation. *Note.* Data from The Lord Corporation, Erie, PA.

the company's health management framework.) According to Robert Penzkover, director of employee benefits at Quaker Oats, "The company's medical care costs had nearly tripled between 1971 and 1981, with Quaker experiencing a 56% increase in the 2 most recent years alone. Within months we instituted a series of cost-control strategies in an attempt to slow future cost increases.

Overall, I think our cost-control success in the past few years is due to three major components. First, our health incentive plan (HIP) was implemented in 1983 to replace our original benefits and give employees a bigger financial stake in the cost and utilization of their medical benefits. To date, it has contributed significantly to lower health costs" (see Figure 2.12). "Second, the 'Informed Choices' program has helped employees and dependents understand their health care options and empowered them with cost, provider, and quality-oriented information to help them make responsible health care decisions. Third, Quaker is counting on health improvement to reduce medical cost increases in the long run as well as decrease disability income claims and increase employee productivity. The company's 'Live Well—Be Well' health promotion program includes health risk appraisals and feedback through questionnaires and clinical screenings; behavioral modification programs in areas such as nutrition, exercise, stress management, substance abuse prevention, smoking cessation, and disease management; and conversion of on-site nurse's clinics to more comprehensive health resource centers to assist employees on a wide range of physical and mental health matters. Although Quaker

Table 2.3
Health Management Personnel and Key Responsibilities
of The Quaker Oats Company

Health management directors	Primary functions
Director, Employee Benefits	Administers health incentive plan (HIP), "Informed Choices," and all health benefit plans
Director, Health & Safety	Administers health promotion, occupational safety, and environmental health programs

Note. Data from The Quaker Oats Company, Chicago, IL.

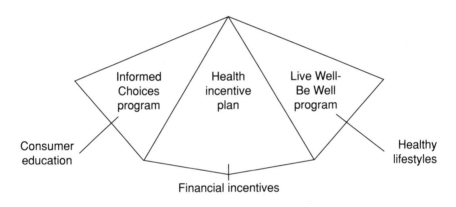

Figure 2.11   The 3-part health management strategy at The Quaker Oats Company. *Note.* Data from The Quaker Oats Company, Chicago, IL.

has offered health promotion programs to employees at some locations for many years, the renewed emphasis formally incorporated the concept into its health management strategy for all areas of the company" (personal communication, 1992).

How Important Is Health Promotion?

For health promotion programs to successfully complement other cost-control strategies, they must achieve certain objectives. First, worksite health promotion efforts must reduce employees' health risks, especially

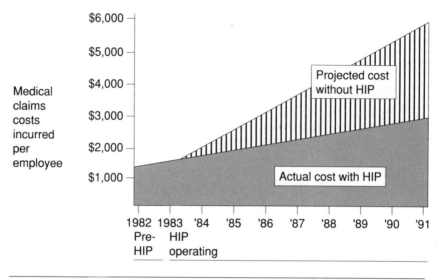

Figure 2.12 Comprehensive medical claim costs incurred before and after the introduction of the health incentive plan (HIP). *Note.* Data from The Quaker Oats Company, Chicago, IL.

smoking, hypertension, high blood cholesterol, musculoskeletal stress, and exposure to carcinogens, all of which can cause early disease, disability, or death.

Second, health promotion activities must help consumers (employees, dependents, and retirees) to clearly understand their health care benefits and motivate them to use health care services properly, especially frequent health care users. To significantly affect specific claims and cost categories, health promotion programs and policies must involve dependents and retirees as much as possible because these two groups typically use about twice as many health care dollars as employees. In a recent survey of 20 randomly selected companies, dependents and retirees used more health care dollars than employees in 18 of the 20 worksites (Chenoweth, 1993).

Third, health promotion efforts must target the most common, most expensive types of health care claims. To do so, decision-makers must closely review an organization's health care data to detect problem areas. Because data reports can vary greatly in format, length, and clarity, decision-makers should request specific types of data from their insurer or claims administrators:

- Institutional inpatient—indicating hospital charges and number of claimants for stays of at least 24 hours for each diagnostic category

- Professional inpatient—indicating charges and number of claimants for medical care, equipment, surgery, anesthesia, and medication for each diagnostic category
- Institutional outpatient—indicating charges and number of claimants for stays of less than 24 hours for each diagnostic category
- Professional outpatient—indicating charges and number of claimants for physician services
- Physician-specific—indicating which doctors and medical facilities were used and the number of claimants using each

Ideally, these profiles should include percentage comparisons between employees and dependents to show usage and costs in all claim categories (see Table 2.4). Thus, program planners can customize specific risk-reduction and health promotion programs for the appropriate target group.

To reduce major claims and costs, health management personnel should analyze the available data and plan appropriate programs and strategies. For example, if an organization's health claims data reflect a high incidence of circulatory, musculoskeletal, and pregnancy-related conditions, program planners should customize specific programs and policies for these problems areas:

Most Common Claims	*Programs and Strategies*
1. Circulatory	<ul><li>Fitness programs</li><li>Smoke-free environment</li><li>Hypertension screening</li><li>Lunchtime sessions on nutrition</li><li>Healthy heart entrees on the cafeteria menu</li></ul>
2. Musculoskeletal	<ul><li>Prework stretching</li><li>Work-hardening exercise for low back, wrist, elbow, key muscle groups</li><li>Ergonomic modifications at work stations</li></ul>
3. Pregnancy-related	<ul><li>Prenatal health education, including screening, drug education, exercise, nutrition</li></ul>

Finally, health promotion programs and policies should be tailored closely to the various interests of employees and dependents. Thus, an

Table 2.4
Sample Health Care Claims Report—Institutional Outpatient Charges by Diagnostic Category (January 1–December 31, 1992)

Diagnostic category	Charges	Percent of charges		Number of claimants	Percent of claimants		Amount paid
		Actual	Norm		Employee	Dependent	
Circulatory system	$ 4,112.50	3.7	4.5	45	43	57	$ 3,500.78
Pregnancy-related	7,430.78	14.5	5.2	19	20	80	6,993.00
Neoplasms	15,000.00	7.8	4.6	15	45	55	13,900.45
Musculoskeletal	4,045.98	4.5	7.8	9	75	25	3,500.00
Injury & poisoning	2,000.00	2.0	3.2	8	0	100	1,500.00
Respiratory system	7,890.00	13.3	9.0	9	10	90	6,578.00

organization should consider which of the following components will appeal to both groups and provide favorable results:

Healthy Lifestyle Education

- Exercise and physical fitness
- Low back care
- Nutrition
- AIDS education
- Prenatal education
- Smoking cessation
- Self-care
- Substance awareness and abuse prevention
- Stress management
- Weight control

Health Care Consumerism

- Health care cost awareness
- Health insurance and benefits education
- Prudent health care usage incentives

Screenings, Monitoring, and Follow-Up

- Cancer screening (breast self-exams, testicular self-exams, colorectal screening)
- Diabetes, blood pressure, and glaucoma screening
- Heart disease risk identification
- Immunizations (e.g., tetanus booster)

Safety Promotion and Accident Prevention

- First aid and cardiopulmonary resuscitation (CPR)
- Choke-saving techniques
- Emergency first aid
- On-the-job safety instruction
- "Right to Know" education (hazardous substances)
- Seat belt and shoulder strap use

Employee Assistance Program

- Alcohol and other drug abuse prevention and treatment
- Mental health counseling
- Domestic counseling (finances, family issues, etc.)
- Preretirement planning

Establishing a Health Management Framework

In planning a health management framework to achieve maximum results, an organization should develop corporate health management goals that are realistically attainable, determine if existing health management personnel have the skills needed to achieve each goal, establish job responsibilities related to each goal, and establish an organizational structure or framework to enhance interpersonal and interdepartmental communication and teamwork.

An integrated health management approach offers employers the greatest opportunity to achieve their goals. For example, many companies have strategically integrated their health promotion activities with a more visible division such as human resources, enhancing visibility, credibility, and administrative support (see Figure 2.13). In essence, such integration provides daily opportunities for personnel in each department (wellness center, medical center, and psychological services) to communicate and work collectively in accomplishing key health management goals. Nevertheless, companies with a multilayered hierarchy, such as Coors, have a unique challenge to ensure that specific decision-making channels are clearly delineated between and among all departments. Job responsibilities must be more clearly defined and performed with less duplication of effort. For instance, an occupational health nurse does a basic health screening on a new employee and detects poor low-back flexibility. Based

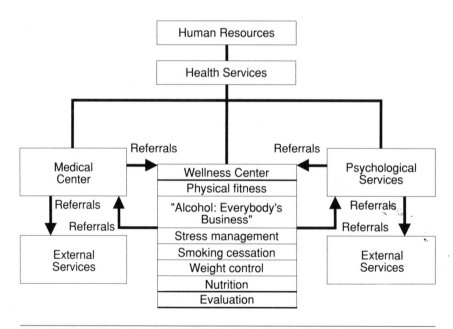

Figure 2.13 The integrated health management framework used at the Adolph Coors Company. *Note.* From *Planning Health Promotion at the Worksite* (2nd ed) (p. 166) by D. Chenoweth, 1991, Dubuque, IA: Brown & Benchmark. Copyright 1991 by Brown & Benchmark. Reprinted by permission.

on this information, the nurse may decide to meet with the personnel or human resources manager to discuss appropriate job opportunities within the employee's capabilities, refer the new employee to an exercise specialist to improve flexibility, or possibly encourage the new employee to participate in the company's prework low-back program. These interventions can improve the employee's low-back health, thus helping the company avoid a preventable injury or accident at the worksite.

In summary, health promotion and other health management interventions must be as closely integrated as possible to have a sustained economic impact at the worksite. Organizations must provide adequate resources, corporate support, and environmental settings for health management personnel to work together. Though a growing number of American companies are benefiting from such integrated efforts, *all* American companies should begin similar efforts in order to stay competitive in the coming years.

References

Bernacki, E., Tsai, S., & Reedy, S. (1986). Analysis of a corporation's health care experience: Implications for cost containment and disease prevention. *Journal of Occupational Medicine, 28*, 502-506.

Busch, R. (1989). Be sure your employees understand their health benefits. *Business & Health, 7*, 36-37.

Business & Health. (1990, April). The 1990 National Executive Poll on Health Care Costs and Benefits, pp. 25-38.

Chenoweth, D. (1991a). Impact of integrated health management frameworks on corporate health care costs. Unpublished manuscript.

Chenoweth, D. (1991b). *Planning health promotion at the worksite* (2nd ed.). Dubuque, IA: Brown & Benchmark.

Chenoweth, D. (1993). *Health care cost management: Strategies for employers* (2nd ed.). Dubuque, IA: Brown & Benchmark.

Penzkover, R. (1984). Building a better benefit plan at Quaker Oats. *Business & Health, 2*, 33-37.

Chapter 3

Using Cost as a Health Promotion Outcome: Problems With Measuring Health in Dollars

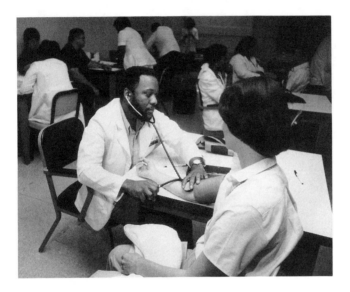

Wendy D. Lynch

Increasing evidence points toward a positive relationship between health-enhancing behaviors and lower health costs (Lynch, Teitelbaum, & Main, 1992; Peterson, 1992; Yen, Edington, & Witting, 1991). This is welcome news to health promotion and human resource professionals who are facing tough decisions about how to control health care expenses. In light of this, it will be tempting for our profession to rely on general, sweeping statements about the cost benefits of a health-oriented lifestyle. Why not? The differences in average costs lead us to such conclusions. For example, smokers alone cost $228 to $878 more a year than nonsmokers (Peterson,

1992; Yen, Edington, & Witting, 1991), good reason to believe that health-compromising behaviors lead to increases in some costs.

What is the catch? Given the well-designed studies that demonstrate the economic benefits of positive health habits, why should we be cautious or skeptical about the evidence we have seen? There are three reasons. First, health care costs more accurately measure use of health services than health status. Second, even if it were a more accurate measure of health status, the cost variable itself is a difficult variable to work with methodologically (Lynch, Teitelbaum, & Main, 1991). Third, health promoters, in general, tend to have a limited understanding of the true nature of health care costs, what influences them, and how to interpret or evaluate them appropriately.

This chapter goes beyond the usual comparisons of overall costs. By examining patterns of health care utilization, it addresses the many possible implications of cost differences between groups. It also introduces a paradigm designed for using and interpreting health claims and examines some of the issues that may help to decipher the health claims puzzle.

Health Care Costs as an Outcome Measure

Health care cost containment is one of the primary goals of worksite health promotion. Consequently, it is no surprise that health care costs often serve as the outcome measure to determine effectiveness of the health promotion program. What should surprise us are the implications of using health care costs as an outcome, although they are not an ideal measure of health status. Indirectly, a company may want healthier employees, but specifically, the company wants less costly employees. These are not the same outcome.

Figure 3.1 presents a simplified view of the desired economic consequences of health promotion on health care costs. The presumed mechanism follows this logic: Health promotion leads to improved current health status. Improved health status leads to reduced likelihood of disease. And reduced risk of disease leads to fewer expenses. Thus, health promotion lowers health care costs.

Obviously, health status and health costs have some relationship, especially in the extreme case. Hospitalization for a terminal condition costs more than treatment in a doctor's office for a minor condition. Similarly, treating a severe fracture probably costs more than treating a minor sprain. But as two conditions become more similar, or more difficult to diagnose, the cost differences become progressively *less* health related. Two identical back problems could have drastically different costs, depending on a complex range of decisions.

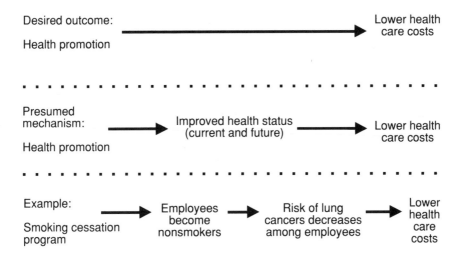

Figure 3.1   The traditional model of how health promotion programs affect costs.

The reverse argument is even less convincing. Would we feel comfortable drawing conclusions about someone's health, just by knowing his or her overall costs? If women average $500 dollars a year more in health costs than men, how valid is the conclusion that men are in better health? Dollars alone provide little indication of personal health status. Yet, health promotion has been willing to stake much of its reputation on dollars alone.

Though they certainly measure health status in some cases, costs often reflect the beliefs, behaviors, and choices of the patient or physician. If we make a list of the constructs that health care costs reflect, it would include, at a minimum, all of the constructs listed in Table 3.1. Many circumstances influence whether employees make contact with the health care system and how they continue that interaction. For convenience we can categorize these circumstances into four general areas: health status and behaviors, health perceptions, the health care system, and health care coverage. Each of these areas shown in Table 3.1 involves several constructs, some of which could fall into more than one category.

Health status accounts for only a portion of the variability in costs. Thus traditionally defined health promotion may also have a limited impact on costs. Indeed, previous research found that *health age* (or *appraised age*), as predicted by a health risk appraisal (HRA), accounted for about 6% of the variability in retrospective health claims (Golaszewski, Lynch, Clearie, & Vickery, 1989). This alone should raise questions about the validity of using insurance claims to assess the impact of health promotion.

Table 3.1
What Health Care Costs Measure

Cost category	Contributing factors
Health status and behaviors	Health status Health-enhancing behavior Health-compromising behavior Intentional conditions (e.g., pregnancy) Family history (inherited health risks) Bad luck
Health care system	Accessibility of service Availability & choice of physicians, specialists, or other health practitioners Geographical region Technological advancement Economics
Health perceptions	Health perceptions Health beliefs (e.g., self-efficacy) Health services-seeking behavior Social & cultural influences
Health care coverage	Health care coverage & benefits Knowledge of benefits

Pieces of the Health Claims Puzzle

As the field of health promotion develops new methods of evaluating and documenting its impact (Lynch et al., 1992; Peterson, unpublished data; Yen, Edington, & Witting, 1991), it becomes more important to understand the different issues that influence health costs, specifically, if we believe that good health behaviors translate into lower costs, why don't low-risk individuals always cost less than high-risk individuals? Why are the cost differences between smokers and nonsmokers greater at Company A than Company B? There are no simple answers to these questions, but understanding some general concepts can lead us to better explanations. At some level, health care costs measure each of four areas.

Health Status and Behaviors

Health status has the most obvious relationship to cost. In theory, the sicker you are, the higher your medical bills. In general this rule probably holds. However, there are exceptions. The previously asymptomatic person who dies of a sudden heart attack probably will have lower health care costs than the person who suffers and survives a slightly less serious heart attack. Health care for a generally healthy person who suffers only from bad luck (e.g., being struck by lightning) will cost more than that for a more fortunate counterpart. Some natural, healthy choices, such as starting a family, also create a need for additional services and, therefore, cause higher costs.

The premise of health promotion is that certain behaviors will influence future health status and thus future health costs. In this light, preventive care becomes an investment whose return will be realized in the future. As mentioned earlier, much evidence supports a relationship between risk behavior and future medical costs. However, we also know that risk awareness often leads to increased health care expenses. Indeed, considering preventive services, greater immediate costs could actually be an indicator of good or improving health rather than poor health.

Another variable in the health risk equation is family history. Family history should and does influence costs by changing the intensity of need for preventive care or screening. Immediate costs for these individuals reflect, not current health status, but their greater likelihood (or fear) of poor health status in the future.

Health Care System

A great deal of the variability in costs lies in the health care system itself or in the patient's choice of where to interact with the system. Small-area analysis studies have demonstrated tremendous differences from one town to the next in the likelihood of patients' undergoing a given medical procedure for the same condition (Wennberg & Gittelson, 1982). Similarly, hospitalizations for similar conditions cost almost twice as much in Boston as in New Haven, Connecticut (Wennberg, Freeman, Shelton, & Bubolz, 1989). The availability of a new, high-tech treatment, such as auto-bone marrow transplant for treatment of breast cancer, will produce costs much higher for the patient who can obtain it than for a patient who does not have access to the procedure (Gale, Armitage, & Dicke, 1991). Choice of type of physician also affects cost. For example, treatment by a specialist is more expensive than treatment by a family physician (C. Cangialose, personal communication, April 24, 1992). Again, these cost differences do not reflect differences in health status.

Obviously, patient choices about when and where to seek medical care will influence cost as well. Interestingly, the greater the inconvenience (e.g., the farther one must drive), the less likely one is to seek care (Simons, Calonge, Kent, & Marshall, 1991). Whether choosing a generalist or a specialist, the emergency room or a local clinic, treatment by a nurse practitioner or a gynecologist—each choice affects the bill.

Health Perceptions

Perceptions about personal health status also influence employee use of health services. The number of times patients visit their physicians corresponds more closely to their personal perception of health than to their physicians' evaluation. For two groups rated equally healthy, those who perceived themselves in poor health averaged 2.4 more visits to their physicians in 1 year than did those who considered themselves to be in good health (Connelly, Smith, Philbrick, & Kaiser, 1991).

Perhaps even more complex are personal beliefs about what might influence health. People who have confidence in modern medicine may have a greater tendency to seek or demand care than those who have less confidence. Similarly, those who doubt their own ability, or self-efficacy, to manage a chronic condition will seek health care services more frequently than those who have confidence in their skills (Lorig & Holman, 1989). Again, these issues affect costs without affecting health.

Preventive behaviors are closely tied to personal beliefs about the value of prevention and one's ability to successfully maintain the behavior. Thus, future health costs will be influenced indirectly by beliefs that enable or discourage an individual from practicing healthy behaviors.

Health Care Coverage

Some variation in costs is due to differences in health care coverage. We know, for instance, that some health services are avoided more often when they are not covered (i.e., paid for) by health insurance or when the employee must bear more of the cost (e.g. cost sharing; Hertzlinger & Schwartz, 1985). Furthermore, employees' knowledge of their benefits may influence their behavior. In the simplest case, someone unsure about coverage may seek certain types of care less frequently than someone who knows the cost will be covered. Obviously this will have more influence on treatment of minor conditions or conditions of less immediate concern.

Companies frequently use benefits redesign as a cost-containment strategy. This is because the amount of the deductible, or the extent of coverage, will influence some health care utilization behaviors especially regarding less serious or less urgent health care needs. Obviously, health care coverage will influence overall health costs. However, its influence on costs—in the short term—has no relationship to health status, only to utilization behavior.

Why Investigate These Factors?

Because overall costs are potentially influenced by all of these factors, they are probably not the appropriate measure of the costs specific to health risk behavior. How, then, should we proceed in examining and understanding costs? Do we narrow our measure to more accurately reflect current health promotion activities, or do we broaden our definition of health promotion to fit the outcome measure (i.e., lowered costs) that has been provided for us? The general call for economic justification of health promotion points out that much of our interest is not necessarily in improving health status but in lowering costs. If so, quantifying the interaction of health-compromising behaviors and health care costs could become our single most important research endeavor.

One way to determine the true relationship between health risks and health costs is to examine only the costs of conditions that have a scientifically proven risk factor. For instance, the costs of smoking might be tied only to the costs of treating lung cancer or other respiratory or cardiovascular consequences of smoking. The cost of not wearing a seat belt would be tied to the actual costs of automobile injuries. (It is less clear how this method would assist in estimating the costs of influences with less understood health implications, such as the role of stress or diet in cancer.)

This approach, now being used by some researchers (Peterson, unpublished data), probably provides the cleanest estimates of risk-cost relationships because it measures specific, identifiable cost areas. These selected cost areas more closely represent true economic consequences than do overall costs. Thus, they reduce interference from all the other possible influences listed in Table 3.1. Clearly this approach provides a better measure of the true cost of health status changes associated with lifestyle.

Despite advances in our ability to identify and isolate more appropriate measures of the economic impact of health promotion, such narrowness of focus could actually impair our view of the big cost picture. As we become more exact in our scientific definition of which diseases health promotion programs can influence in the future, we become more precise in one dimension but not necessarily more informed overall. It is unlikely that the impact of health promotion will be limited to those outcomes that have been documented in the health literature. This approach leaves out the other questions such as, what influence does health promotion have on health care utilization behavior?

We know that adopting healthy behaviors can influence many more dimensions of utilization than future health status. Health promotion programs may influence employees' attitudes, their likelihood of seeking care, even their choice of health care provider. These in turn will influence costs, perhaps even more quickly than any change in health status. Our understanding of each of these constructs will help untangle the pieces and position health promotion within a comprehensive health management approach.

Why should we be interested in all of these areas when strong evidence has begun to verify the economic value of health promotion? Presenting a simplified view of the relationship between health risk and costs without acknowledging the complexity of health care utilization behavior is both misleading and counterproductive to the long-term survival of health promotion. If we choose to live by the dollar, we must understand its limitations and learn from them.

Thus, in order to advance, we must choose between two paths: either more precise measures of cost or a broader perception of what influences costs. Although we have not acknowledged our arrival at this fork in our profession's road, the path we choose will have a great impact on the future role and definition of health promotion. We may choose to establish a credible, precise economic model that justifies current health promotion efforts. Or we may choose to redefine health promotion to include the many variables involved in an individual's decision to seek health care services.

Costs Not Associated With Health Status

To understand these concepts, we need only take notice of existing cost differences that cannot be explained easily based on health status alone. The following observations were obtained through a detailed analysis of diagnosis-specific data. Results are not described in detail but only as an illustration of the concepts introduced here.

Gender Differences

Generally, men have lower health care costs than women (Lynch, Gillfilan, Jennett, & McGloin, 1993). Some of the difference stems from child-bearing costs and more periodic exams, which begin at a younger age for women than for men. However, women also have greater relative costs for diagnoses such as mental health, skin problems, and upper respiratory problems. Men have greater costs for ischemic heart disease and hypertension. From the traditional health promotion viewpoint, men have more risk factors and should cost more on average. But they don't, even when we remove child-bearing costs. It is difficult to attribute this to health status differences.

Utilizing Information From HRAs

The complexity of costs is perhaps best illustrated by one phenomenon that does not follow our usual expectations about health risks and costs. Studies of two separate employee populations suggest that HRA responders are more likely to use medical services than employees who do not take the HRA (Lynch, Gillfilan, Jennett, & McGloin, 1993; Lynch, Golaszewski, Clearie, & Vickery, 1989). The more recent of these studies also examined the health risk levels of the two groups. As has been reported in other studies, HRA responders had lower levels of health risk in virtually all categories (Nice & Woodruff, 1990). They also reported fewer known health problems and better perceived health status overall. From all logical indications, the HRA group had fewer reasons to seek care and should have needed fewer health care dollars. Why then, did the HRA responders use more services and have higher costs, on average, than nonresponders?

Several observations suggest that there are distinct health care utilization differences between those who responded to the HRA and those who did not. (Recall that the HRA responders perceived themselves to be in better health and, as a group, had fewer risk factors.) For example, HRA nonresponders were more likely to avoid the medical system altogether (see Figure 3.2). Men and women nonresponders were two and

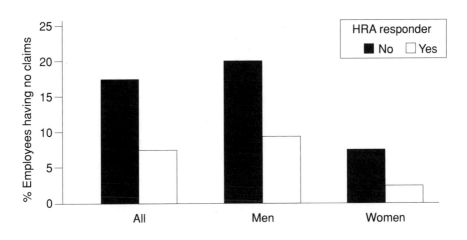

Figure 3.2   Employees who did not respond to the HRA were consistently less likely to use medical services. This difference was evident for both male and female employees. Interestingly, the HRA responders had fewer health risks and perceived themselves in better health. (The data reflect 1988 and 1989 health care costs.)

three times more likely, respectively, than responders to have no medical claims.

HRA responders were more likely to seek care for a given problem. HRA responders sought care for common diagnoses more frequently than nonresponders (see Figures 3.3 a & b). These included both chronic and acute conditions. For women, the cost for these 10 diagnoses was $459 a person over 2 years. For men, 10 common diagnoses accounted for an additional $61 a person. These differences cannot be due to overall health status alone.

HRA responders were more likely than nonresponders to seek some specialized services. For example, they were almost twice as likely to seek eye care than nonresponders. Was this due to perceived health risk or to knowledge of benefits?

HRA responders were more likely to seek ongoing care for certain conditions such as mental health problems, chiropractic care, hypertension, and allergies. Responders averaged more visits for a given problem than nonresponders. Could this reflect a difference in attitude toward self-management of a problem?

HRA responders seemed more likely to undergo preventive services than HRA nonresponders. Given that HRA responders initiated more frequent contact with the health care system, some of this difference could reflect either efforts to prevent problems in the future or increased awareness of preventive care. Could it also reflect the "worried well" syndrome (Lynch et al., 1993)?

None of these observations have simple explanations. Health status and health risk differences certainly do not help us understand them. In fact, these utilization patterns contradict our expectations based on established health promotion convictions. The cost differences reflect some influence other than, or in addition to, health status or risk. Perhaps *all* of the factors in Table 3.1 play a part.

Certainly, there is a pattern of increased utilization by those who choose to seek health information through the HRA, though an explanation for this phenomenon will not emerge from estimates of the relationship between health status and cost. That is to say, if we stay too narrow in our focus, the precision will actually make us less informed.

It should be noted that the health plan at this company covered many services that are not covered by other plans. Consequently, the differences in costs detected here may not appear under other plans. In addition, this company rewarded HRA respondents by lowering the copayment from 15% to 10%. HRA respondents could have been better aware of their benefits or simply more highly motivated to use them. Nonetheless, these individuals had lower health risks but used health services more.

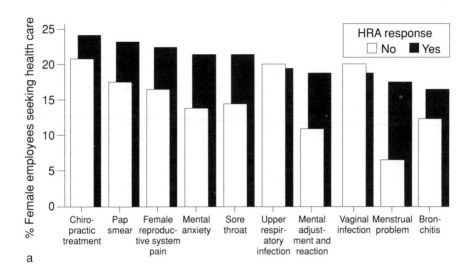

a

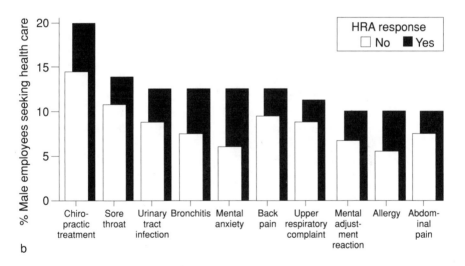

b

Figure 3.3 (a) Female HRA responders were more likely than non-responders to seek care for 8 of 10 most common diagnoses and procedures. Nonresponders sought care more often for upper respiratory and vaginal infections. (The data reflect 1988 and 1989 health care costs.) (b) Male HRA responders were more likely than nonresponders to seek care for all of the top 10 most common diagnoses. (The data reflect 1988 and 1989 health care costs.) *Note.* Data from "Health Risks and Health Insurance Claims Costs: Results for Health Hazard Appraisal Responders and Non-Responders" by W.A. Lynch, L.A. Gilsillan, C. Jennett, and J. McGloin, *Journal of Occupational Medicine*, *35*(1), pp. 28-33.

Summary

Much of the credibility of health promotion in the corporate arena rests on its proven economic value. Accordingly, our field has accepted health care costs as one of its primary outcome measures. We have also accepted the premise that improved health status will be measurable in terms of lower health care expenses.

The hazard in this argument is in accepting costs as a reasonable indicator of health status. Health care costs reflect an individual's degree of contact with and intensity of use of health care resources. Although some of these behaviors are health related, others are not. Indeed, health promotion could have a dramatic impact on health status that is obscured by other cost components. More importantly, a substantial portion of health care costs have nothing to do with health status. Thus, the greatest opportunities for cost containment, our accepted outcome, may rest outside the usual health promotion strategies.

If we truly want to understand use of health services, we must understand all of the factors that influence use. Suppose adopting a health enhancing behavior saves $50 a year in reduced disease and adds $30 a year in requested services. Obviously, we are detecting (and celebrating) the $20 net reduction in costs. But we also have a $30 opportunity. Perhaps the $30 spent might be reduced further by medical self-care, policy changes, or education. What makes an HRA responder more likely to seek care or to seek more comprehensive care? The answers may lead to a more inclusive role for health promotion in the future.

Now that we have jumped collectively onto the economic bandwagon, we must resist the temptation to limit our field to a simple, unidimensional model of how health promotion affects health costs. The interactions of the many factors that determine costs are anything but simple.

References

Connelly, J.E., Smith, G.R., Philbrick, J.T., & Kaiser, D.L. (1991). Healthy patients who perceive poor health and their use of primary care services. *Journal of General Internal Medicine, 6*, 47-51.

Gale, R.P., Armitage, J.O., & Dicke, K.A. (1991). Autotransplants: Now and in the future. *Bone Marrow Transplantation, 7*, 153-157.

Golaszewski, T.J., Lynch, W.D., Clearie, A., & Vickery, D.M. (1989). The relationship between retrospective health insurance claims and a health risk appraisal-generated measure of health status. *Journal of Occupational Medicine, 31*(3), 262-264.

Hertzlinger, R.A., & Schwartz, J. (1985, July). How companies tackle health care costs: Part I. *Harvard Business Review*, pp. 69-81.

Lorig, K., & Holman, H.R. (1989). Long-term outcomes of an arthritis self-management study: Effects of reinforcement. *Social Science Medicine*, **29**(2), 221-224.

Lynch, W.D., Gillfilan, L.A., Jennett, C., & McGloin, J. (1993). Health risks and health insurance claims costs for health hazard appraisal responders and nonresponders. *Journal of Occupational Medicine*, **35**(1), 28-33.

Lynch, W.D., Teitelbaum, H.S., & Main, D.S. (1991). The inadequacy of using means to compare medical costs of smokers and non-smokers. *American Journal of Health Promotion*, **6**, 123-129.

Lynch, W.D., Teitelbaum, H.S., & Main, D.S. (1992). Comparing medical costs by analyzing high-cost cases. *American Journal of Health Promotion*, **6**(3), 206-213.

Lynch, W.D., Golaszewski, T.J., Clearie, A., & Vickery, D.M. (1989). Characteristics of self-selected responders to a health risk appraisal: Generalizability of corporate health assessments. *American Journal of Public Health*, **79**(7), 887-888.

Nice, D.A., & Woodruff, S.I. (1990). Self-selection in responding to a health risk appraisal: Are we preaching to the choir? *American Journal of Health Promotion*, **4**(5), 367-372.

Simons, L.A., Calonge, B.N., Kent, C.G., & Marshall, G. (1991). Relationship between distance traveled for labor and delivery care and adequacy of prenatal care for women residing in rural Colorado counties. *Clinical Research* (abstract), **39**(1), 30A.

Wennberg, J., Freeman, J., Shelton, M., & Bubolz, T. (1989). Hospital use and mortality among medicine beneficiaries in Boston and New Haven. *New England Journal of Medicine*, **321**, 1168-1173.

Wennberg, J., & Gittelson, A. (1982). Variations in medical care among small areas. *Scientific American*, **246**, 120-134.

Yen, L.T., Edington, D.W., & Witting, P. (1991). Associations between health risk appraisal scores and employee medical claims costs in a manufacturing company. *American Journal of Health Promotion*, **6**(1), 46-54.

PART II

Assessment and Evaluation

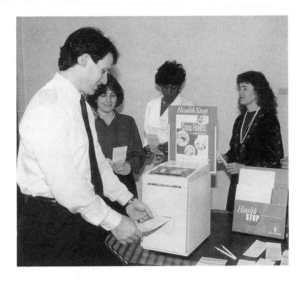

Identifying the economic impact of worksite health promotion must necessarily be considered within the construct of broader measurement and evaluation issues. This section discusses the important factors that must be considered when developing program evaluation strategies and how cost-benefit analysis and cost-effectiveness analysis must often be dovetailed within this broader framework.

One important method for understanding the impact of worksite health promotion is cost-effectiveness analysis. In chapter 4, Marc Schaeffer, Anastasia Snelling, Maura Stevenson, and Robert Karch review the methods employed to determine the effectiveness of health promotion programs in reducing health risk. They give particular attention to the use of health risk appraisal instruments as tools for measuring risk reduction. They then look at some important cost factors, such as absenteeism, productivity, and health care utilization, and review the effects—both positive and negative—of worksite health promotion interventions on those factors. Finally, the authors review some of the methodological difficulties imposed by the realities of evaluation in the work setting.

Chapter 5 provides a useful road map for designing and implementing an effective program evaluation. Steve Hoover, Marilyn Jensen, Robert Murphy, and David Anderson carefully define the nature of program evaluation and its enhancement of the decision-making process. They then take the reader step-by-step through an effective evaluation, including how to avoid roadblocks to implementing necessary changes.

Two important sources of data for measuring the effectiveness of worksite health promotion are insurance claims and employee survey data. In chapter 6, Jeffrey Harris and Kenneth Theriault provide useful tools for capturing data relevant to program effectiveness. Most organizations have the necessary insurance claims and other sources; however, finding and arranging data into a usable format is often a monumental task. The authors give important recommendations on which data are useful and how to interpret their reliability and validity.

Chapter 4

Worksite Health Promotion Evaluation

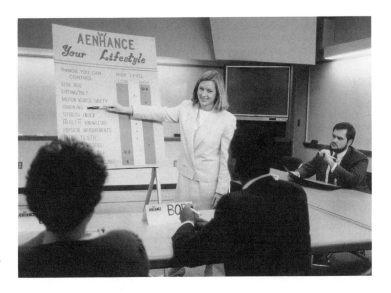

Marc A. Schaeffer
Anastasia M. Snelling
Maura O. Stevenson
Robert C. Karch

With no apparent relief in sight from rising health care costs, and with many corporate benefits packages in danger of reduction or elimination, many U.S. companies have turned to health promotion as a possible solution to an escalating problem. Despite the increase in popularity of these health promotion programs and the cost-saving suggestions from several worksite health promotion (WSHP) evaluation studies, many critics argue that the benefits neither balance nor outweigh the costs. However, the present enthusiasm for health promotion in American society is concurrent with awareness of the nation's health care crisis and a direct by-product of the nation's health status. Soaring health care costs are fueling debate on national health insurance and cost containment. In 1990, costs topped $671 billion, and accounted for 12.2% of the gross national product (Gladwell, 1991; U.S. Bureau of the Census, 1990).

The economic burden associated with poor health and premature death in the United States is staggering, with a particular burden on organizations. Corporations pay more than 28% of the health care bill (Loomis, 1989). In a pessimistic forecast, Herzlinger and Schwartz (1985) predicted that if health care costs are not contained, they could consume corporate profits by 1993. Thus, it is no mystery that many corporations have been involved more with the direct action of WSHP than as bystanders to political opinion and public debate.

Although many large and small corporations alike have adopted WSHP strategies, it is not clear whether these programs have been effective in achieving the desired cost-cutting goals. Further, although a growing body of literature indicates that WSHP has been instrumental in helping employees reduce health risks, and consequently aiding employers in averting costs, there has been debate as to whether these positive outcomes have been validly measured and evaluated.

We present here a review of several major worksite health promotion studies and the variety of results that have been reported, focusing on effectiveness. As a preface, we summarize the definition of WSHP and its evaluation. Although dozens of articles have been published on WSHP evaluation during the last 20 years, the emphasis of the evaluations has varied. Moreover, studies have been performed in different regions of the country, using participants from diverse business settings, and executed with different research methodologies. These variations in time, region, setting, and method have been both a strength and a weakness. We conclude our chapter with a review of the current state of WSHP research and suggestions for possible improvements that could meet critics' concerns.

Defining Health Promotion

Many definitions of health promotion have been suggested over the years, though in terms of promotion, the emphasis has been on the optimization of health rather than the prevention of disease (O'Donnell, 1986). Optimal health includes improved intellectual functioning, physical fitness, emotional fitness, energy levels, coping ability, and lowered risk of disease (Everly & Feldman, 1985). In a more recent definition of health promotion,

Green and Kreuter (1991) state that health promotion is "the combination of educational and environmental supports for actions and conditions of living conducive to health" (p. 4). This concise statement reflects the recent tendency toward inclusion of social as well as individual responsibility for health, and facilitation of individual behavior change in tandem with organizational and social change approaches to health promotion (Green & Kreuter, 1991).

Numerous histories and retrospectives on the origins and goals of WSHP (Jacobson, Yenney, & Bisgard, 1990; Sloan, Gruman, & Allegrante, 1987; Terborg, 1986) reflect its evolution and its place within American corporate culture. Kiefhaber and Goldbeck (1983) characterized this development as representing four generations of WSHP. The first generation of programs was closely related to health protection and safety, whereas second-generation programs concentrated on a single health issue, such as hypertension or obesity. Despite the advances of more comprehensive third-generation programs, which included screening individuals for appropriate specialized interventions, these past programs never fully transcended the individual as recipient of program benefit. However, the fourth-generation approach goes beyond mere coordination of health programs to the complete integration of health promotion into all aspects of work life, including personnel, hiring, job placement, occupational safety, medical services, and numerous other areas of the work situation. Current WSHP efforts and program changes suggest that fourth-generation WSHP programs are already taking shape in organizations preparing for the work force of the 1990s.

Evaluating Health Promotion at the Worksite

Escalating health care costs have motivated organizations to assess the value of health promotion strategies in light of a broader organizational performance perspective. Despite the commonly held belief that WSHP makes good "business sense" (for a variety of reasons, including the cost-control aspects previously discussed), there has been considerable demand for data that prove the effectiveness and benefits of these programs. However, several surveys indicate that the majority of companies that sponsor health promotion programs do not conduct any type of evaluation (Christenson & Kiefhaber, 1988; O'Donnell, 1988; Warner, Wickizer, Wolfe, Schildroth, & Samuelson, 1988).

Similarly to other types of evaluation, WSHP evaluation is performed for reasons of program justification, improvement, effectiveness, or continuation. At its most basic level, an evaluation portrays the program in terms of attendance, facility usage, and participation rates. Evaluation of program effectiveness can include much greater intricacy: Program outcomes such as screening results, changes in risk factors, remarkable case histories, or changes in measures of organizational performance (e.g., absenteeism, productivity, and retention) may be examined. Effectiveness results are often presented in relation to cost of implementation or cost-effectiveness analysis. Perhaps the most complicated level of evaluation involves the ascription of monetary value to program outcome measures. Commonly known as cost-benefit analysis, this level of evaluation provides results that are both promising and controversial. The promise of cost-benefit analysis suggests that WSHP in the management of corporate human capital could enormously enhance worker and organizational potential. The results are controversial because of the nonstandard methodologies, which cast doubt on how findings have been generated (O'Donnell, 1988).

Although WSHP appears to be achieving its goal of reducing the health risks that affect the work force, WSHP may affect other important organizational elements, with health risk reduction being the springboard. These elements include reductions in absenteeism, increases in productivity, and control over health claims costs. It is not a coincidence that these four elements—health risk, absenteeism, productivity, and health care cost—are the measures most frequently analyzed in WSHP evaluation research. However, to reemphasize the theoretical perspective of WSHP-induced change, lower health risk is the precursor to positive effects in other areas.

Reducing Health Risks

The evolution of health promotion programs has paralleled societal focus on disease prevention through lifestyle management. This has created a need for a means of assessing individual modifiable behaviors and health risks. Furthermore, a quantification of health risk both for individuals and groups has become desirable for purposes of identification and screening, education, and evaluation. The health risk appraisal, to a large extent, serves these purposes for many health promotion programs. Generally, HRAs take the form of self-report questionnaires but are often integrated with selected clinical and physiological measures. The HRA is a health promotional tool that emphasizes cardiovascular risk and is used to enhance awareness of health risks and their associated lifestyle behavior patterns. HRAs normally compare individual behaviors and personal characteristics with epidemiological data to estimate the probability of a client's dying within a specified time period. Figure 4.1 shows a segment of the popular HRA developed by the Carter Center of Emory University.

Health risk appraisal is an educational tool. It shows you choices you can make to keep good health and avoid the most common causes of death for a person your age and sex. This health risk appraisal is not a substitute for a check-up or physical exam that you get from a doctor or nurse. It only gives you some ideas for lowering your risk of getting sick or injured in the future. It is NOT designed for people who already have HEART DISEASE, CANCER, KIDNEY DISEASE, OR MOST OTHER SERIOUS CONDITIONS. If you have any of these problems and you want a health risk appraisal anyway, ask your doctor or nurse to read the report with you.

DIRECTIONS: Your answers will be treated as confidential. To get the most accurate results, answer as many questions as you can and as best you can. If you do not know an answer, leave it blank. Questions with a ★ (star symbol) are important to your health, but are not used by the computer to calculate your risks. However, your answers may be helpful in planning your health and fitness program.

Please put your answers in the empty boxes.   (Examples: ☒ or ☐125☐)

1. Sex	1 ☐ Male 2 ☐ Female
2. Age	☐ Years
3. Height (Without shoes) (No fractions)	☐ Feet ☐ Inches
4. Weight (Without shoes) (No fractions)	☐ Pounds
5. Body frame size	1 ☐ Small 2 ☐ Medium 3 ☐ Large
6. Have you ever been told that you have diabetes (or sugar diabetes)?	1 ☐ Yes 2 ☐ No
7. Are you now taking medicine for high blood pressure?	1 ☐ Yes 2 ☐ No
8. What is your blood pressure now?	☐ / ☐ Systolic (high no.) / Diastolic (low no.)
9. If you *do not* know the numbers, check the box that describes your blood pressure.	1 ☐ High 2 ☐ Normal or low 3 ☐ Don't know

(continued)

Figure 4.1 Healthier People Health Risk Appraisal. This appraisal, developed by the Carter Center of Emory University, is one example of a commonly used HRA. This HRA questionnaire asks about both life-style habits and physiological data. Accompanying software for this HRA computes an individual's probability of dying in the next 10 years from 42 different causes. Moreover, the software algorithm converts an individual's health risk into a key variable known as health age. *Note.* From Computer Outfitters, (800) 827-2567.

10. What is your TOTAL cholesterol level (based on a blood test)?	[_____] mg/dl
11. What is your HDL cholesterol (based on a blood test)?	[_____] mg/dl
12. How many cigars do you usually smoke per day?	[_____] cigars per day
13. How many pipes of tobacco do you usually smoke per day?	[_____] pipes per day
14. How many times per day do you usually use smokeless tobacco? (Chewing tobacco, snuff, pouches, etc.)	[_____] times per day
15. CIGARETTE SMOKING How would you describe your cigarette smoking habits?	1 [ ] Never smoked ☞ Go to 18 2 [ ] Used to smoke ☞ Go to 17 3 [ ] Still smoke ☞ Go to 16
16. STILL SMOKE How many cigarettes a day do you smoke? ☞ GO TO QUESTION 18	[ ] Cigarettes per day ☞ Go to 18
17. USED TO SMOKE a. How many years has it been since you smoked cigarettes fairly regularly? b. What was the average number of cigarettes per day that you smoked in the two years before you quit?	[ ] Years [ ] Cigarettes per day
18. In the next 12 months, how many thousands of miles will you probably travel by each of the following? (NOTE: U.S. average = 10,000 miles) a. Car, truck, or van: b. Motorcycle:	[ ] ,000 miles [ ] ,000 miles
19. On a typical day how do you USUALLY travel? (Check one only)	1 [ ] Walk 2 [ ] Bicycle 3 [ ] Motorcycle 4 [ ] Sub-compact or compact car 5 [ ] Mid-size or full-size car 6 [ ] Truck or van 7 [ ] Bus, subway, or train 8 [ ] Mostly stay home

Figure 4.1 *(continued)*

20. What percent of the time do you usually buckle your safety belt when driving or riding?

☐ %

21. On the average, how close to the speed limit do you usually drive?

1 ☐ Within 5 mph of limit
2 ☐ 6-10 mph over limit
3 ☐ 11-15 mph over limit
4 ☐ More than 15 mph over limit

22. How many times in the last month did you drive or ride when the driver had perhaps had too much alcohol to drink?

☐ Times last month

23. How many drinks of alcoholic beverage do you have in a typical week?

☞ (MEN GO TO QUESTION 33)

(Write number of each type of drink)
☐ Bottles or cans of beer
☐ Glasses of wine
☐ Wine coolers
☐ Mixed drinks or shots of liquor

WOMEN
24. At what age did you have your first menstrual period?

☐ Years old

25. How old were you when your first child was born?

☐ Years old
(If no children write 0)

26. How long has it been since your last breast X-ray (mammogram)?

1 ☐ Less than 1 year ago
2 ☐ 1 year ago
3 ☐ 2 years ago
4 ☐ 3 or more years ago
5 ☐ Never

27. How many women in your natural family (mother and sisters only) have had cancer?

☐ Women

28. Have you had a hysterectomy?

1 ☐ Yes
2 ☐ No
3 ☐ Not sure

29. How long has it been since you had a pap smear?

1 ☐ Less than 1 year ago
2 ☐ 1 year ago
3 ☐ 2 years ago
4 ☐ 3 or more years ago
5 ☐ Never

Figure 4.1 *(continued)*

★30. How often do you examine your breasts for lumps?	1 ☐ 2 ☐ 3 ☐	Monthly Once every few months Rarely or never
★31. About how long has it been since your had your breasts examined by a physician or nurse?	1 ☐ 2 ☐ 3 ☐ 4 ☐ 5 ☐	Less than 1 year ago 1 year ago 2 years ago 3 or more years ago Never
★32. About how long has it been since you had a rectal exam? ☞ (WOMEN GO TO QUESTION 34) MEN	1 ☐ 2 ☐ 3 ☐ 4 ☐ 5 ☐	Less than 1 year ago 1 year ago 2 years ago 3 or more years ago Never
★33. About how long has it been since you had a rectal or prostate exam?	1 ☐ 2 ☐ 3 ☐ 4 ☐ 5 ☐	Less than 1 year ago 1 year ago 2 years ago 3 or more years ago Never
★34. How many times in the last year did you witness or become involved in a violent fight or attack where there was a good chance of a serious injury to someone?	1 ☐ 2 ☐ 3 ☐ 4 ☐	4 or more times 2 or 3 times 1 time or never Not sure
★35. Considering your age, how would you describe your overall physical health?	1 ☐ 2 ☐ 3 ☐ 4 ☐	Excellent Good Fair Poor
★36. In an average week, how many times do you engage in physical activity (exercise or work that lasts at least 20 minutes without stopping and that is hard enough to make you breathe heavier and your heart beat faster)?	1 ☐ 2 ☐ 3 ☐	Less than 1 time per week 1 or 2 times per week At least 3 times per week
★37. If you ride a motorcycle or all-terrain vehicle (ATV), what percent of the time do you wear a helmet?	1 ☐ 2 ☐ 3 ☐ 4 ☐	75% to 100% 25% to 74% Less than 25% Does not apply to me
★38. Do you eat some food every day that is high in fiber, such as whole grain bread, cereal, fresh fruits, or vegetables?	1 ☐ Yes 2 ☐ No	

Figure 4.1 *(continued)*

★39. Do you eat foods every day that are high in cholesterol or fat, such as fatty meat, cheese, fried foods, or eggs?   1 ☐ Yes   2 ☐ No

★40. In general, how satisfied are you with your life?
1 ☐ Mostly satisfied
2 ☐ Partly satisfied
3 ☐ Not satisfied

★41. Have you suffered a personal loss or misfortune in the past year that had a serious impact on your life? (For example, a job loss, disability, separation, jail term, or the death of someone close to you.)
1 ☐ Yes, 1 serious loss or misfortune
2 ☐ Yes, 2 or more
3 ☐ No

★42a. Race
1 ☐ Aleutian, Alaska native, Eskimo, or American Indian
2 ☐ Asian
3 ☐ Black
4 ☐ Pacific Islander
5 ☐ White
6 ☐ Other
7 ☐ Don't know

★42b. Are you of Hispanic origin such as Mexican-American, Puerto Rican, or Cuban?   1 ☐ Yes   2 ☐ No

★43. What is the highest grade you completed in school?
1 ☐ Grade school or less
2 ☐ Some high school
3 ☐ High school graduate
4 ☐ Some college
5 ☐ College graduate
6 ☐ Post graduate or professional degree

Figure 4.1   *(continued)*

Although administration of HRAs is normally efficient and cost effective relative to a complete medical assessment (Warner et al., 1988), use of the HRA has stimulated discussions of its validity and reliability. It is virtually impossible to make a statement about HRAs in general because there is much variability among the dozens of HRAs in use. However, examination of the more widely used instruments demonstrates favorable validity and reliability results.

The use and reported benefits of HRAs continues to expand and in some cases are exaggerated (Wagner, Beery, Schoenbach, & Graham, 1982). However, their use seems to be an integral part of more comprehensive health promotion efforts. In a recent survey of 1,358 worksites, 24.1% reported using an HRA as part of their health promotion activities. The perceived benefits included improved employee health, increased productivity, and reduced health care costs (Office of the Assistant Secretary for Health and the Surgeon General, 1979).

The HRA also serves as an evaluation instrument for many studies that attempt to determine cost-effectiveness and cost benefit. Its ability to quantify health risk through the generation of several key variables makes it well suited for such studies. Both health age, also known as appraised age, and health index are calculated variables that reflect an individual's level of health risk relative to a calculated standard. *Health age* is actuarially based, expressing the risk of dying relative to a cohort matched in age and gender; *health index* reflects the magnitude of the difference between health age and actual age. A favorable health age is lower in value than an actual age, and the greater the positive difference between actual age and health age, the more favorable the health index (see Figure 4.2).

Participant A—Favorable Health-Age Rating
    Age (years)   37
    Health Age (years)   33
    Health Index   4

Participant B—Unfavorable Health-Age Rating
    Age (years)   37
    Health Age (years)   41
    Health Index   −4

Figure 4.2 Hypothetical illustration of favorable and unfavorable health age and health index calculation. Two hypothetical examples for different participants who have completed a health risk appraisal are shown. Participants are the same age, but participant A has a favorable health-age rating and participant B has an unfavorable health-age rating. The health age has been calculated by an algorithm within the health risk appraisal that assigns weights for individual HRA questions, so such factors as advanced age or smoking contribute to poorer ratings and such factors as regular exercise habits or a negative family history for cardiovascular disease allow for a more favorable health-age outcome. Note that participant A exhibits a favorable health age (i.e., actual age is older than the health age). The opposite is true for participant B, whose actual age is younger than the health age. Moreover, the sign for health index is positive for participant A and negative for participant B.

Measuring Health Risks

Several WSHP studies report significant health risk reduction. Though there is wide variation in study factors, such as length of study, content of program exposure, and variables examined, there are changes in the health risk variable, a desired outcome measure of health promotion programs.

In one of the earliest studies to examine changes in health risk, Rodnick (1982) followed 292 employees of Optical Coating Laboratories who participated in the HRA program and received educational materials. Participants underwent a baseline HRA and a 12-month retest. Health age of male employees decreased over this period. At baseline, the average health age for men was 0.60 years less than chronological age, and at the end of 12 months, 2.37 years less than chronological age. Women showed an average initial health age of 1.32 years less than chronological age, and after 1 year showed an average health age of 1.58 years less than chronological age. The change in average health age for women was not significant.

Another study sought to determine the effect of participation in exercise on health risk. Following 616 males at CIGNA Corporation for 12 months, DeLucia, Goodspeed, Goldfield, and Beltz (1986) found differences in health risk change based on exercise participation level. Highly active participants (those who exercised two or more times a week) maintained their risk level (disease rate of 4.6 per 100) over the course of the year. In terms of statistical risk, the highly active participants offset the aging factor during that year. In comparison, the moderately active, marginally active, and inactive groups saw an increase in their risk of heart disease.

In two separate studies, health age decreased following participation in a comprehensive health promotion program, despite the passage of 6 months. A 1/2-year decrease in health age occurred among 426 Army staff participants who were tested at program entry and at the 6-month follow-up (Karch et al., 1988). Because this reduction occurred over 6 months, it was expressed as the change attributed to health age plus the intervening time. In effect, participants manifested a 1-year reduction in health age. Additionally, the greatest improvement in health age and health risk occurred in those who had the highest participation rate in the health promotion program. These results corroborate those of an earlier study conducted at the Toronto Assurance Company. Shephard, Corey, and Cox (1982a) found that after 6 months, a control group had a mean increase in health age of 0.48 years. Because age should have increased by 0.5 years concurrently with the calendar year, Shephard interpreted this as a net 0.02 gain in appraised age of extended life years. Using the same principle, high adherents to the fitness program experienced a net gain of 1.26 years compared to low adherents who only had a 0.45 net gain.

Other researchers have studied a variable similar to health age. At Blue Cross/Blue Shield of Ohio, researchers examined the health risk index for participants and controls in the intervention modules (controls were individuals who had also filled out HRA questionnaires). At posttest, participants in the physical conditioning module at Blue Cross/Blue Shield of Ohio scored more favorably in health risk than the control group. The health risk index was significantly improved for participants in nutrition and weight-control components, but participants in stress management and smoking cessation modules did not exhibit any appreciable change in health risks (Conrad, Riedel, & Gibbs, 1988). The researchers suggested that this effect was possibly mediated by an increased level of fitness training among participants in nutrition and weight-control components.

Golaszewski and co-authors (1989) used the health risk index to examine the relationship between HRA data and 3 years of retrospective health insurance claims data at The Travelers Insurance. The premise that a higher health risk index (which could represent an indirect measure of health status) correlates with a lower rate of medical utilization held true for men but not for women. In another study, the relationships between 18 health-related measures in an HRA (including risk index) and medical claims costs of 1,838 employees were examined for 3 consecutive years. A strong statistical relationship was found between positive health behaviors and lower medical claims, regardless of age and sex, for 11 measures (Yen, Edington, & Witting, 1991).

AT&T Communications employees were offered a health promotion program that incorporated an HRA developed by General Health, Inc. This HRA included a job- and health-related attitudinal survey developed specifically for this study. Data included blood pressure, lipid profile, Type A-behavior profile, alcohol consumption, and exercise habits as well as the standard questions for coronary artery disease (CAD) and cancer risk. Though some participants completed an HRA plus intervention modules, one control group participated only in an HRA, whereas another group was offered neither an HRA nor intervention. The program participants showed increased levels of exercise, decreased smoking levels, improved overall perception of individual health, reduced CAD risk, and reduced overall mortality over the next 10 years. Although there were some improvements among individuals who completed only an HRA, *no* benefits were observed in the group that had been offered no intervention opportunities (Spilman, Goetz, Schultz, Bellingham, & Johnson, 1986).

In a similar study (Faust et al., 1983), employees of Blue Cross/Blue Shield of Michigan were divided into four groups, each of whom were variously exposed to health promotion activities. The group that received the most comprehensive exposure to activities, such as an HRA, screening, group and individual counseling, and risk reduction programs, experienced significant improvement in productivity, health attitudes, and health risks when compared to groups who received less exposure.

Few studies have attempted to put an economic value on health promotion-induced changes in health risk. Karch et al. did so in a 1988 study of Army staff. Over the course of the 3-year study, 4.8 lives were computed to have been saved for this group. Because the value of an employee to an organization was assumed to be twice the average loaded salary ($53,789), a net benefit of $516,374 was realized from averted mortality. In the study conducted at Toronto Assurance, Shephard et al. (1982a) applied a benefit of $37.90 per worker-year to the positive changes in health risk.

Although HRAs help researchers identify prominent risk factors, assign employee risk ratings for health benefits, and motivate behavioral change resulting in risk reduction, there are a few difficulties with this commonly used WSHP tool. The variety of HRAs creates one type of difficulty; the research methods associated with administering an HRA has generated other questions. Finally, despite several attempts to assess the economic impact of reductions in health risk, just how one should do so is still unclear.

Reducing Absenteeism

Worker absenteeism has long been of interest and concern to organizations. The number of lost work days and the subsequent cost to businesses are staggering. The economic impact of worker absenteeism derives from direct and indirect costs. Direct costs include the decreased productivity of absent workers and less experienced replacements and the additional expense of hiring substitute labor. Indirect costs include productivity losses caused by other workers supervising substitute labor and spending time away from their own jobs to perform the tasks of absent workers (Howard & Mikalachki, 1979). These indirect costs can be 3 to 6 times the direct costs (Bowne, Russell, Morgan, Optenberg, & Clarke, 1984).

The issues surrounding absenteeism in the workplace are not well understood. Reviews of the extensive literature on absenteeism (Breaugh, 1981; Muchinsky, 1977) indicate that this is due in part to a dearth of consistent, valid measures of absenteeism. Muchinsky (1977) reported over 41 measures of absenteeism. Such variety of measurement has "clouded the exact meaning of many studies that investigated the relationship between absenteeism and other variables" (p. 317).

For many organizations, the connection between health promotion programs and absenteeism is based on the contention that healthy employees are sick less often (Hoffman & Hobson, 1984). Thus, it follows that programs that have been shown to improve employee health via weight reduction, smoking cessation, exercise and physical conditioning, or the enhancement of job satisfaction may lower the absentee rate. The large number of reports documenting the effects of WSHP on absenteeism is evidence of the intense interest among businesses in managing this persistent problem.

Relating Absenteeism and Measures of Activity

Although a variety of relationships have been studied, the primary focus of literature regarding WSHP and absenteeism has been on the relationship between exercise and absentee rates. One classic study in England by Linden (1969) investigated the relationship between maximal oxygen uptake ($\dot{V}O_2$max) and absence from work for customs officers, fire fighters, and office workers. Linden found an inverse relationship between $\dot{V}O_2$max and the number of sick leave absences among customs officers, although no such relationship was found among fire fighters and office workers. The data provided no explanation for the lack of relationship, but Linden did suggest that the effects of exercise on $\dot{V}O_2$max for fire fighters (specifically, the increase of maximum aerobic power) would be minimal because of the higher baseline fitness levels required by their occupation. Without exception, comparisons of exercisers with nonexercisers have yielded the same finding: exercisers use less sick leave (Bjurstrom & Alexiou, 1978; Blair et al., 1986; Faust et al., 1983; Gettman, 1986; Horowitz, 1987; Karch et al., 1988; Pender, Smith, & Vernof, 1987; Reed, 1985; Shephard, Cox, & Corey, 1981). For example, exercisers at Tenneco Corporation used about 36 hours of sick time annually compared to 45 hours for nonexercisers (Baun, Bernacki, & Tsai, 1986).

In a study conducted at Mesa Petroleum, Gettman (1986) also found a significant difference of 1.5 days of sick leave between fitness program participants and nonparticipants, who were employed by Mesa for both the control year and the study year. An interesting substudy examined attendance of those employees who changed exercise status during the 2 years. Though the sample size was too small and variable for significance, changes in absenteeism were charted uniformly in the expected direction. Employees who became sedentary during the study year increased their use of sick leave during the same time period. Those who became exercisers in the study year used less sick leave than they did in the control year. Though the associations between exercise and absenteeism are encouraging, it has been difficult to determine what influence selection biases have on the observed differences between exercisers and nonexercisers.

Selection bias was examined at a study conducted at The Travelers Insurance worksite fitness center. Employees who joined the center had a history of fewer absences due to illness even before the study began (Lynch, Golaszewski, Clearie, Snow, & Vickery, 1990). Yet members experienced significantly fewer absences in 1988 compared to 1986; nonmembers did not. Controlling for gender and previous absences, members could be expected to have 1.2 fewer absences than nonmembers. In other words, members began the program having an advantage over nonmembers, and membership in the program further increased the difference in sick leave use between the two groups.

When exercisers are assessed by amount of regular exercise, the relationship between exercise and absenteeism becomes more pronounced. In a study of a Canadian company, Cox and Shephard (1979) found that high adherents (i.e., those who exercised the most) initially demonstrated the same absentee rate as other employees but experienced a 22% lower rate after 6 months. Gettman's study (1986) at Mesa Petroleum looked at activity levels measured in kilocalories per kilogram of body weight per week and demonstrated that as caloric expenditures rose, the absentee rate fell.

At Blue Cross/Blue Shield of Ohio, researchers showed that as frequency of vigorous exercise increased, short-term absenteeism due to illness decreased significantly. This translated to approximately 1 less day of absenteeism a year for each regular exerciser compared to nonexercisers (Conrad et al., 1988). Lynch et al. (1990) also documented a reliable negative correlation between members' participation rates and the number of absences from work at The Travelers Insurance.

In these studies, absenteeism was correlated to the level of participation in exercise and fitness programs. Participation reflects exposure to a health promotion program, but it cannot be assumed that a high adherent is highly fit or that a low adherent is poorly fit. Several studies have examined the relationship between measures of physical fitness and employee absenteeism.

Relating Absenteeism and Measures of Fitness

Blair et al. (1986) examined absenteeism among Dallas educators before and after exposure to a health promotion program. Those who completed the program had an average of 1.25 days less absenteeism during the study year than nonparticipants. Improvement in physical fitness, measured by increased treadmill time, had a significant association with reduced absenteeism. This link between a change in status (presumably due to the health promotion program) and absenteeism strengthens the inference that reduction in absenteeism among participants was a result of the program.

More recently, the work of Tucker, Aldana, and Friedman (1990) examined the extent of the relationship between absenteeism and cardiovascular fitness. Subjects were 8,301 employees of corporations nationwide that participated in a health screening program. Absenteeism due to illness in the last 6 months was self-reported. Controlling for age, gender, income, smoking, and percent body fat, a strong inverse association between sick leave and fitness level was demonstrated. Subjects in the poor fitness group had 2.5 times the rate of high absenteeism (defined as absences of 5 or more consecutive days) compared to those in the excellent fitness category.

Many researchers have found a gender difference in absentee rates. Tucker et al. (1990) showed that females reported more illness absences than males, and the association between the cardiovascular fitness and absenteeism was stronger for females than for males. Baun et al. (1986) found that both exercising and nonexercising females had higher absenteeism rates than their male counterparts, findings that have been corroborated in other studies (Gettman, 1986; Horowitz, 1987; Karch et al., 1988).

Relating Absenteeism and Comprehensive WSHP Interventions

Many investigations of the influence of WSHP on absenteeism have examined programs that offer a comprehensive array of interventions. In addition to exercise, these may include smoking cessation, nutrition education, weight control, hypertension detection, stress management, and other education modules.

Studies that examined the extent of participation in health education (i.e., classroom-based) components of a health promotion program revealed similar trends. The Federal Highway Administration utilized a 2-year pre- and posttest design to determine the effect of a health promotion program on absenteeism (Horowitz, 1987). Sick leave data on 42 participants for 12 months before and 12 months after program implementation were examined, revealing a significant decrease in absenteeism of 14.7 hours for each participating employee (26.4%).

An evaluation of the comprehensive TriHealthalon Program at General Mills (Wood, Olmstead, & Craig, 1989) compared the rate of absenteeism (1 year before program initiation, 1984, to 1 year after) between 685 participants and 341 nonparticipants from the sales division. Their data showed a statistically significant increase of 69% in absenteeism from 1984 to 1985 for nonparticipants, whereas participants' absenteeism showed a decrease of 19% for that period.

A study of the absenteeism experience of two groups of Johnson & Johnson employees over a 3-year period was reported by Jones, Bly, and Richardson (1990; see also chapter 11). Employees at four company sites where a comprehensive health promotion program had been introduced were compared with employees at five company sites without the health promotion program. Among wage earners, adjusted mean levels of absence among the health promotion participants were found to decline over the study period and were significantly lower than mean absence levels for nonparticipants. No significant differences were found for salaried personnel.

Resulting Value of Absenteeism Reduction

Numerous researchers have assigned a monetary benefit to absenteeism reduction. Most recently, a pre- and posttest control group design was used at DuPont Company (Bertera, 1990). Forty-one intervention sites and 19 control sites employing 29,315 and 14,573 full-time hourly workers, respectively, provided data on annual mean number of disability days per hourly worker (disability being a measure of absenteeism that includes all illnesses not related to occupational causes). Employees at intervention sites demonstrated a 14% decline in disability days over 2 years; employees at control sites showed a decrease of 5.8%. This difference amounts to 11,726 fewer disability days at program sites over 2 years, or a $1,596,877 savings. These savings, based on the cost of wages, compensation, and benefits, were enough to offset program costs (including one-time start-up costs) in the first year. That year, every dollar spent on health promotion yielded $1.10 in lower disability costs. In the second year the return was $2.05; the average return on investment was $1.42.

Karch et al. (1988) examined pre- and posttest intervention sick leave use records for 535 participants in the Pentagon's ARSTAF program. Sick leave recorded for 9 months before participation in the health promotion program was compared to the amount of sick leave recorded for the 9 months after participation. Participants exhibited a significant decline of 5.9 hours during the postparticipation period. Furthermore, nonparticipants used sick leave more during the same period. Though participants were exposed to the health promotion program for only 12 weeks, and the researchers used a conservative approach to calculating the financial benefit of reduced sick leave, a net benefit of $534,554 was realized.

In the Dallas Independent School District, annual absenteeism was reduced by 1.25 days a person for 2,546 participants. Based solely on the cost of substitute teachers ($47 a day), this reduction yielded actual savings of $149,578 (Blair et al., 1986). Reed, Mulvaney, Billingham, and Skinner (1986) investigated the relationship between absence hours due to illness of participants versus nonparticipants and a comprehensive health promotion program at Blue Cross/Blue Shield of Indiana from 1978 to 1982. Savings of $180,000 were reported.

In 1979, when the costs of paid absenteeism (excluding holidays, vacation, unpaid absenteeism, and disability) were measured at Blue Cross/Blue Shield of Michigan (Faust et al., 1983), the savings were $28,951. Based on the average net real hourly wage (cost of labor including medical and dental insurance, FICA, and workers compensation) discounted to the appropriate year, annual savings in the years 1981 and beyond were $33,067. The total net present value of benefits saved because of reduced absenteeism in this study group was $190,979. A similar measurement of disability absences showed a reduction in disability hours worth a net present value gain of $23,987.

Leave usage is the measure commonly used in health promotion research. However, because of the complex theoretical association between health promotion and absenteeism and the limitations of research and methodology, definitive causal links between health promotion and leave reduction are not yet firmly established.

Increasing Productivity

Productivity is a component of performance, not a synonym for it, and therefore is only one of a number of performance criteria useful in evaluations (Sink, Tuttle, & DeVries, 1984). As our economy evolves from one based on manufacturing into one based on service and information, there is a concomitant need to accurately measure white-collar productivity. Research and development, logistics, strategic planning, and personnel are all areas in which whole projects may be placed on time lines and evaluated. However, for the white-collar employees of these departments, there are no widgets being produced, and no set number of sales calls to be made. In short, very few readily quantifiable and uniformly accepted measures of job performance exist.

WSHP is seen as a way to enhance employee productivity. Unlike typical productivity enhancement techniques, exercise and behavior change programs create unique opportunities for interaction among employees from all levels and functional areas, thus affecting core organizational values (Terborg, 1986). Falkenberg (1987) presented a model that showed how knowledge-worker (i.e., white-collar) job performance could be enhanced via exercise. He found that the physiologic arousal levels of individuals who exercise regularly may be more appropriate than those of less fit individuals for executing cognitive tasks. The physically fit individual's more rapid dissipation of physiological tension—that is, better stress resistance—leads to improved productivity. Also, the availability of fitness facilities at work gives employees greater flexibility in scheduling work and nonwork activities. With management support that allows workers to take exercise breaks from their cognitive tasks, productivity could approach maximum.

Measuring Productivity

Several studies of white-collar productivity and WSHP failed to provide statistically significant data, yet demonstrated encouraging results. Shephard et al. (1981), working with Canada Life, and Bernacki and Baun (1984) at Tenneco employed supervisory ratings to evaluate the impact of 6-month and 12-month exercise programs on productivity and attitudes. There were gains in productivity for participants as well as for controls at Canada Life. At Tenneco, there was a positive association between above-average job performance and increasing levels of exercise. Edwards and Gettman (1980) saw similar results when they studied the real estate commissions of sales personnel who participated in a progressive 12-week aerobic exercise program. Although there was no statistically significant difference between experimental and control groups, there was a tendency in the exercising group toward increased physical fitness and increased sales.

In the Army staff project, productivity improvement was measured by using the employee's self-evaluation questionnaire with a parallel supervisory evaluation. Participants were allowed 3 hours of work time a week to participate. All other factors being equal, time away from work could have caused a productivity decline. However, there was no indication of a decline. Though the results were not statistically significant, the findings showed that whereas nonparticipants reported themselves to be declining in productivity and participants reported a steady level, supervisory ratings showed a decline among nonparticipants but an *increase* among participants (Karch et al., 1988).

Extrapolating Productivity From Attitudinal Change

Because it is extremely difficult to measure white-collar productivity changes, investigators have focused their efforts on assessing the attitudinal effects of WSHP, though this, too, is difficult (Grana, 1985; Rudman, 1987). The link between attitude, or morale, and productivity was explicated by Howard and Mikalachki (1979), who described two major pathways by which WSHP might affect short-term and intermediate-term productivity. They asserted that an employee's participation in an exercise program or fitness improvement leads to changes in attitudes and feelings as well as in levels of energy. In turn, these changes affect productivity through the employee's ability to work longer and more efficiently in the office, improved loyalty and job satisfaction, and commitment to the company.

Investigators have often used surveys and interviews to quantify morale, job satisfaction, and related attitudinal elements. Durbeck et al. (1972) administered questionnaires to participants 6 months and 12 months after they entered NASA's fitness program. Of those members who exercised three or more times a week (high adherents), 90% reported better health and greater stamina, and nearly 50% felt that their work performances improved. Rhodes and Dunwoody (1980) and Yarvote, McDonagh, Goldman, and Zuckerman (1974) similarly surveyed regular participants of worksite exercise programs for their subjective response to the program's effects. Subjects reported an increased sense of well-being, an improved capacity for sustained physical effort, and improved self-confidence and outlook on the job.

Spilman and colleagues (1986) evaluated a pilot program at AT&T. Using HRAs that included job-related attitudinal questions and were administered before and after exposure to a wide selection of health education and exercise modules that lasted 4 to 12 weeks, they saw statistically significant improvements in health risk factors, such as reductions in cholesterol, diastolic blood pressure, and Type A behavior. They also reported that employees believed that after their participation in the health modules they were more energetic and their productivity and quality of work life had improved.

Holzbach et al. (1990) investigated the effects of the LIVE FOR LIFE program on Johnson & Johnson employees in four companies that offered the full program over a 2-year period. Three Johnson & Johnson companies comprised a nonequivalent control group. No overall change in attitudes was found on measures of job involvement, growth opportunities, respect from family and friends, or relations with coworkers, but the LIVE FOR LIFE companies recorded significant improvement in attitudes regarding organizational commitment, satisfaction with supervisory relations, working conditions, job competence, pay and fringe benefits, and job security (see chapter 11). All of these attitude measures, except job competence, maintained their significant gains over baseline at Year 1 and Year 2. "The sustained effect over a broad range of attitude measures is thought to reflect the pervasive changes in the organizational environment brought about by implementation of the program" (p. 977).

Not all WSHP programs produce change. In the Johnson & Johnson study, attitudes at one of the LIVE FOR LIFE companies did not improve over the 2-year study period, "suggesting that business conditions and management support may have an equally important effect on the success of change actions" (Holzbach et al., 1990, p. 978). At Signature Corporation, clerical-worker members of the fitness center showed a significant difference in productivity measures, but there were no significant differences in the Index of Job-Related Strain and the State-Trait Anxiety Inventory (Pender et al., 1987). At Liberty Corporation, Blair et al. (1980) used a composite productivity report, incorporating variables on sick leave hours, merit increases, recent promotions, and a supervisor's rating. Their data did not support a consistent relationship between these measures of job performance and exercise.

There are very few credible studies directly linking individual outcomes of WSHP programs with productivity improvements because of the difficulty in quantifying this variable. Therefore, cost-benefit and cost-effectiveness analyses involving productivity are not easily translated. The trend of the research is toward improved measurement of productivity using attitudinal indicators such as job satisfaction and morale.

Controlling Health Care Costs

Health care utilization and the resultant costs are a growing concern among individuals, corporations, and governments. Health care costs in the United States have been rising at a dramatic rate for many years. In 1970, national health care expenditures totaled $75 billion and accounted for 7.4% of the gross national product (GNP). In 1980, those figures increased to $248.1 billion, which reflected 9.1% of the GNP. National health expenditures in 1990 were $671 billion, or 12.2% of the GNP. This is almost double the 6.5% devoted to military expenditures (Gladwell, 1991; U.S. Bureau of the Census, 1990). It is estimated that by the year 2000, the figure will have risen to over $1 trillion (Brennan, 1982).

One of the expressed purposes of WSHP is to lower the absolute need for health care services, while also shifting some portion of that need from costly therapeutic services to less expensive preventive care. However, Herzlinger and Schwartz (1985) found in their survey of large American corporations that although 24% of net profits was expended on health insurance, only 1/10th of 1% was disbursed for health promotion.

The literature abounds with anecdotal evidence of health care cost savings achieved through WSHP programs (Terborg, 1986). In fact, several recent studies using HRA-based data have found strong associations between poor health behaviors and higher medical claims costs (Golaszewski & Lynch, 1988; Yen et al., 1991). Programs intended to lower the need for health care have been implemented by numerous companies, large and small. The savings in health care costs over both the short- and long-term can be substantial.

Influencing Health Care Costs With Fitness Interventions

Several studies have used a cardiovascular and strength-training fitness program as their sole or primary intervention in efforts to control medical costs. Among these is the work of Baun et al. (1986) at Tenneco, which showed annual medical cost savings of $553 a person when comparing exercisers with nonexercisers in a corporate health promotion program. This represented a 48.2% reduction in ambulatory health care costs.

Researchers at The Prudential Insurance Company reported a 45.7% reduction in major medical costs after the first year of an exercise program that also included frequent seminars on lifestyle improvement (Bowne et al., 1984). When adjusted for imbalances in maternity usage, medical costs were still reduced by 37.5% during the same period in which health care costs for the nation were increasing at a rate of 12.5%.

Bowne et al. (1984) also examined the relationship between participation and number of disability days and direct disability costs. The findings confirmed that at 1 year postentry, this cohort experienced a 20.1% reduction in its average use of disability from the year before program entry. Losses from salary continuation during a disability period were reduced by 31.7%, an average savings of $91.24 a participant. The average combined savings (medical plus disability) for each participant was $353.38

compared to an average program operation cost of $120.60 a participant. These results indicate that WSHP programs can make a substantial contribution to the control of health care and disability costs in the short-term.

At GE Aircraft Engines in Cincinnati, Hollenback and Heck (1991) investigated whether employee use of the GE Aircraft Engines' Fitness Center helped control medical costs. Medical claims of approximately 800 members were examined for 6 months before and for 12 months after joining the center. A group of about 2,700 nonmembers served as a comparison group. The two groups were different in that members, before joining the center, had 35% higher mean medical care costs than nonmembers ($1,044 vs. $773 a person, respectively). After joining the center, mean medical care costs dropped to $787 a person for members. These lower costs are due primarily to shorter hospital stays, which, on average, dropped from 5.1 to 3.8 days a year. The control group's costs rose by 22% to $941 a person, which is consistent with medical care cost inflation during the study period. All figures are statistically significant. Conservative estimates of savings include $540,000 in members' medical costs, plus the productivity benefits of avoiding 762 hospital days a year.

At Canada Life, Shephard and colleagues found a 35% increase in medical costs for a control company while a firm with a fitness program saw only a 1% rise overall, which also included a 4.1% reduction in claims by participants considered to be high adherents (Shephard, Corey, Renzland, & Cox, 1982b). At Mesa Petroleum, Gettman (1986) saw a lower annual medical cost of $217 each for participants in their fitness program, though it was not clear if the effect was due to the program itself or to the self-selection of healthier employees as participants.

Patterson (1986), at United Methodist Publishing House, also saw lower annual medical costs of $349 for participants in a multicomponent corporate health promotion program. However, similarly to the Mesa study, whether the desired savings were the result of the program or of biased participant selection was unclear. At Control Data Corporation, researchers found a $1.8 million savings in health care costs based on the comprehensive StayWell Program (Jose, Anderson, & Haight, 1987).

The Army staff project (Karch et al., 1988) did not reveal the expected decrease in participants' health care costs. However, this discrepancy may have resulted from the methodological problems of the small sample size, as well as a large variance in health claims costs. Significant negative correlation was found, though, between $\dot{V}O_2max$ and monetary spending on health claims. Furthermore, participants who logged the most hours had the greatest decrease in number of health services used.

Assessing the Economic Impact of WSHP on Health Care Costs

The benefits of positive change in health behaviors may best be seen in the long term. For this reason, and because the field is relatively new, there have been very few studies demonstrating statistically significant proof of the effectiveness of comprehensive WSHP programs in reducing health care costs (Conrad et al., 1988; Wood et al., 1989). At Johnson & Johnson, researchers assessed health care costs over a 5-year period in a program that offered a wide range of intervention classes in addition to physical conditioning. Two participant groups showed mean annual increases for inpatient services of $43 and $42, versus an increase of $76 for the control group (Bly, Jones, & Richardson, 1986).

Blue Cross/Blue Shield of Indiana, in a long-term study (4.75 years), saw a mean difference in health care costs of 24% between participants and nonparticipants in the company's health promotion program. This translated into a savings of $519 a person during the study (Gibbs, Mulvaney, Henes, & Reed, 1985).

Several studies have projected savings because of WSHP. At The Travelers Insurance, a study covering 1986 to 1990 showed a trend toward increased cost savings for each year of the program. Estimated savings for the 5-year period totaled $24.86 million. In 1990 the savings were $7.82 million. Contributing to this were reductions in unnecessary physician visits ($0.62 million) and decreased emergency room visits ($0.17 million) (Bureau of National Affairs, 1991).

Participants in AT&T's pilot program "Total Life Concept," attained risk reductions in smoking, physical inactivity, and aggregate risk. Based on this data, Bellingham, Johnson, McCauley, and Mendes (1987) estimated that health benefit savings would be $312.2 million over 10 years *if* the Total Life Concept program were to be extended to all 100,000 AT&T employees.

The rapidly rising cost of health care has forced organizations to take a serious look at countermeasures. WSHP is a strategy common to several organizations, which has apparently helped control rising health care costs. Although some studies conducted for a year or less suggest promising results, a long-term study of 4 to 5 years is needed to better indicate probable health savings. Clearly, it takes time to attain health improvements and consequently, there will be a time lag between spending for WSHP and seeing a reduction in health care costs.

Weighing the Results of WSHP Evaluation

Despite the consistent finding that WSHP is effective and that these programs save money, several critics have called attention to the problem of research methodologies. It is true that research methodology has been inconsistent and in many instances lacking in experimental rigor. This lack of consistency in research methods allows for opposing judgments. One can be extremely critical of the findings because results were not generated by a common, rigorous method. Or one could argue that despite the wide variety of approaches, a common theme has emerged. Though it is clear that WSHP evaluation research can be improved, it is also clear that not *all* the existing studies have arrived at faulty conclusions.

Removing Methodological Barriers

The execution of most WSHP evaluations share several common problems (Conrad, Conrad, & Walcott-McQuigg, 1991; Katz & Showstack, 1990; Warner et al., 1988), notably the lack of random selection and assignment of participants. Other methodological deficiencies include nonstandard definition of independent and dependent measures, unknown validity and reliability of questionnaires, and variable retest intervals. Moreover, many WSHP studies have reported significant differences based on small samples, or estimated results, or given hypothetical outcomes. Many studies have used improper statistical tools, and even those that have been subjected to sound analysis fail to acknowledge the statistical power of results.

Many of these methodological shortcomings can be corrected. There are a number of studies, although not using rigid selection and assignment criteria that have made attempts to circumvent this shortcoming. Some longitudinal studies have attempted to use participants themselves as controls and with some success. Moreover, a number of studies have very effectively demonstrated that the degree of positive outcome was directly proportional to the amount of participation time. Unless one can produce data indicating that employees traditionally resistant to participation in WSHP either definitely will not participate or simply do not have the ability to improve, the dose response results from several studies (Karch et al, 1988; Karch et al., 1991; Shephard, 1982b) should be given consideration.

Furthermore, researchers should make an effort to apply WSHP-induced benefits only to those employees who demonstrate the positive changes, rather than generalizing the benefits to the personnel of an entire organization with its complex, heterogeneous demographics. Finally, researchers should acknowledge their primary methodological problems when they draft papers. If authors neglect to mention these idiosyncratic difficulties, critics may conclude that the authors are ignorant of proper techniques or trying to hide something, or both. Of course, it is much easier to be a critic of the existing literature than it is to design and execute the definitive study. Perhaps one of the most important corrections would be better research planning.

Many of the major methodological difficulties in the evaluation of WSHP programs stem from conflicts created by the requirements of traditional social science research: rigorous controls, strict isolation of program elements, long-term follow-up, and the desire to provide a positive service to as wide an audience as possible (Murphy, Gasparotto, & Opatz 1987; Smith, McKinlay, & Thorington, 1987). The ideal or truly scientific WSHP research setting should have no direct or implied conflict between the stated purposes and the logistic feasibility of program implementation. However, many constraints affect the implementation and evaluation of WSHP, including limitations on time, personnel, finances, data availability, and conflicting organizational needs.

Efforts that replicate true experimental design have been the preferred method of research (Cook & Campbell, 1979), but these have not been very successful in the evaluation of WSHP programs. In fact, the true experimental design may not be the appropriate methodology. Murphy et al. (1987) have stated that, "Imitating the techniques of other established sciences can retard the substantive development of worksite health promotion and lead to the compilation of data of less value than otherwise possible" (p. 10). The challenge presented by such inherent methodological issues is not to discard the organizational evaluation of WSHP because of the absence of scientific rigor, but to realize the distinct differences between laboratory research and field research (Murphy et al., 1987). Given such differences, a discussion of methodological issues is necessary, with particular attention to the dependent measures: health risk, sick leave, productivity, and health care utilization.

Refining Measures of Health Risk, Absenteeism, Productivity, and Health Care Costs

Despite their popularity, there has been only limited examination of the validity of HRAs. Moreover, there are literally dozens of both public domain and proprietary HRAs, some having as few as a handful of questions, others having several hundred. Not surprisingly, some HRAs are better predictors of morbidity and mortality than others, those that use the most sophisticated logistic equations being superior (Smith et al., 1987). What is surprising in the literature is the frequent failure to identify which HRA has been used in research. Another notable drawback of most HRAs is the lack of attention to quality of life. The measurement of health risk is an area ripe for standardization, and the credibility of this measure may depend on a stricter definition.

Absenteeism data have been collected through use of company records, personnel files, monthly time-sheets, and, in some cases, self-reports. Because of the numerous company policies regarding legitimate use of sick leave, not all studies purporting to measure sick leave actually measure such leave. Depending on how detailed the leave records are, some researchers have attempted to isolate personal sick leave by excluding identifiable reasons for leave use such as maternity leave, care of sick child, family illness, disability leave use, unpaid sick leave, and scheduled absences such as vacations or holidays (Anderson & Jose, 1987; Bjurstrom & Alexiou, 1978; Chenoweth, 1988; Faust et al., 1983; Van Tuinen & Land, 1986).

A good example of how organizational decisions impose limits on analyses of potential WSHP-dependent measures is found in the policies of Control Data Corporation. Control Data has no sick leave data after 1985 because it initiated a cost-containment incentive into its benefits package, which allowed each employee a specified number of leave days, for any purpose, to be managed by the individual. As a result, sick leave became indistinguishable from vacation or other types of leave (Anderson & Jose, 1987). Clearly, there is ample room for standardization of absenteeism data and the methods used to analyze this important measure.

There are a broad number of psychological and physical factors that have been claimed to affect productivity (Howard & Mikalachki, 1979). Multifactorial influences on dependent measures like productivity often make it hard, if not impossible, to show definitive causal effects. Additionally, because of complex interactions between productivity and other factors (including absenteeism), confirming most operationalizations of productivity are exceedingly difficult.

Numerous definitions and treatments of other common dependent measures, such as health care utilization and costs, also create problems for evaluators of WSHP. There are too many methods by which medical costs are tabulated. Some studies divide costs into physician, inpatient, and outpatient categories (Bernacki, Tsai, & Reedy, 1986), whereas others partition costs according to treatment areas such as orthopedic, gynecological, and obstetric (Shephard et al., 1982a).

Studies that include health care utilization as a dependent measure are difficult to review, particularly considering the diverse elements of benefit programs, such as coverage, copayments, and deductibles. These variations may be useful to corporations in marketing their benefit packages, but they greatly compromise the validity of claims data for research and evaluation. The Federal Highway Administration determined that it was impractical even to collect claims data because of the many insurance-carrier options offered to federal employees as well as the employees' option to change insurance carriers every year (Horowitz, 1987).

The Need for WSHP Evaluation Standards

Assuming one has good data representing health risk, absenteeism, productivity, and health claims, and these measures reveal at least some positive statistically reliable outcomes, it is still a challenge to fit the positive outcomes to a defensible economic impact. For example, if a program has demonstrated that health risk has been reduced sufficiently to claim the saving of 12 lives, what is the economic value of 12 lives? Further, if a program has been associated with reduction in absenteeism and increased productivity, recruitment, retention, and morale, how does one attach an accurate dollar figure to these improvements?

The answers to these questions are not simply found or constructed. Several researchers have grappled with these questions and developed their own unique schemes to assess economic impact. Unfortunately, most, if not all, of the methods that have been used in cost-benefit analysis of WSHP are sufficiently unorthodox that critics trained in economics (and cost-benefit analysis) have a field day finding faults.

Again, this problem of nonuniform economic analyses calls for a standard paradigm. However, not every WSHP research project is amenable to the same rules of analysis, and thus it seems even more imperative to heed the recommendation of O'Donnell (1988). He argues that although leaders of WSHP acknowledge the importance of evaluation of economic impact and cost-benefit analysis, it is probably a poor investment for most employers. Moreover, given the exorbitant cost of doing a good job of WSHP evaluation, this type of research should be done primarily by academe, government, philanthropic organizations, and the pooled resources of interested employers. Additionally, such efforts should be focused only on programs that are known to be top-notch with the necessary data readily available (O'Donnell, 1988).

The "state-of-the-art" in research and evaluation of WSHP has yet to be obtained or defined. All research to date has been affected by many of the methodological problems discussed in this section. Given that the proper research style is still in its early developmental and exploratory stages, users or researchers should use the same caution that Aristotle gave to his Athenian students:

> Therefore in discussing subjects, and arguing from evidence, conditioned in this way, we must be satisfied with the broad outline of truth. . . . for it is a mark of the trained mind never to expect more precision in the treatment of any subject than the nature of that subject permits.
>
> Aristotle,
> *Nicomachean Ethics,*
> Book One

References

Anderson, D.R., & Jose, W.S., II. (1987). Employee lifestyle and the bottom line: Results from the StayWell Evaluation. *Fitness in Business,* **2**(3), 86-91.

Baun, W.B., Bernacki, E.J., & Tsai, S.P. (1986). A preliminary investigation: Effect of a corporate fitness program on absenteeism and health care cost. *Journal of Occupational Medicine*, **28**, 18-22.

Bellingham, R., Johnson, D., McCauley, M., & Mendes, T. (1987). Projected cost savings from AT&T Communications Total Life Concept (TLC) Process. In J.P. Opatz (Ed.), *Health promotion evaluation: Measuring the organizational impact* (pp. 35-42). Stevens Point, WI: National Wellness Institute.

Bernacki, E.J., & Baun, W.B. (1984). The relationship of job performance to exercise adherence in a corporate fitness program. *Journal of Occupational Medicine*, **26**, 529-531.

Bernacki, E.J., Tsai, S.P., & Reedy, S.M. (1986). Analysis of a corporation's health care experience: Implications for cost containment and disease prevention. *Journal of Occupational Medicine*, **28**, 502-508.

Bertera, R.L. (1990). The effects of workplace health promotion on absenteeism and employment costs in a large industrial population. *American Journal of Public Health*, **80**, 1101-1105.

Bjurstrom, L.A., & Alexiou, N.G. (1978). A program of heart disease intervention for public employees—A five year report. *Journal of Occupational Medicine*, **20**, 521-531.

Blair, S.N., Blair, A., Howe, H.G., Pate, R., Rosenberg, M., & Parker, G.M. (1980). Leisure time physical activity and job performance. *Research Quarterly for Exercise and Sport*, **51**, 718-723.

Blair, S.N., Smith, M., Collingwood, T.R., Reynolds, R., Prentice, M.C., & Sterling, C.L. (1986). Health promotion for educators: Impact on absenteeism. *Preventive Medicine*, **15**, 166-175.

Bly, J.L., Jones, R.C., & Richardson, J.E. (1986). Impact of worksite health promotion on health care costs and utilization: Evaluation of Johnson & Johnson's LIVE FOR LIFE Program. *Journal of the American Medical Association*, **256**, 3235-3240.

Bowne, D.W., Russell, M.L., Morgan, J.L., Optenberg, S.A., & Clarke, A.E. (1984). Reduced disability and health care costs in an industrial fitness program. *Journal of Occupational Medicine*, **26**, 809-816.

Breaugh, J.A. (1981). Predicting absenteeism from prior absenteeism and work attitudes. *Journal of Applied Psychology*, **66**, 555-560.

Brennan, A.J.J. (1982). Health promotion: What's in it for business and industry. *Health Education Quarterly*, **9**, 9-19.

Bureau of National Affairs. (1991). Travelers scores $7.8 million in savings from comprehensive program. *Benefits Today*, **8**, 263-264.

Chenoweth, D.H. (1988). The impact of health education on absenteeism in a health care setting. *Fitness in Business*, **2**(4), 133-136.

Christenson, G.M., & Kiefhaber, A. (1988). Highlights from the national survey of worksite health promotion activities. *Health Values*, **12**(2), 29-33.

Conrad, K.M., Conrad, K.J., & Walcott-McQuigg, J. (1991). Threats to internal validity in worksite health promotion program research: Common problems and possible solutions. *American Journal of Health Promotion*, **6**(2), 112-122.

Conrad, K.M., Riedel, J.E., & Gibbs, J.O. (1988). The effect of the Blue Cross and Blue Shield worksite health promotion programs on employee absenteeism. (Final Report to the W.K. Kellogg Foundation Project Number UHMD0001AL). Chicago: Health Services Foundation.

Cook, T.D., & Campbell, D.T. (1979). *Quasi-experimentation: Design and analysis for field settings*. Chicago: Rand McNally.

Cox, M.H., & Shephard, R.J. (1979). Employee fitness, absenteeism and job satisfaction. *Medicine and Science in Sports and Exercise*, **11**, 105.

DeLucia, A., Goodspeed, R., Goldfield, N., & Beltz, S. (1986). Health promotion at CIGNA. *Corporate Commentary*, **2**(2), 13-24.

Durbeck, D.C., Heinzelmann, F.K., Schacter, J., Haskell, W.L., Payne, G.H., Moxley, T., III, Nemiroff, M., Limoncelli, D.D., Arnoldi, L.B., & Fox, S.M. (1972). The National Aeronautics and Space Administration—U.S. Public Health Service health evaluation and enhancement program. *The American Journal of Cardiology*, **30**, 784-790.

Edwards, S.E., & Gettman, L.R. (1980). Determining the value of employee fitness programs. *Personnel Administrator*, **25**(11), 41-44, 61.

Everly, G.S., & Feldman, R.H. (1985). *Occupational health promotion: Health behavior in the workplace*. New York: Wiley.

Falkenberg, L.E. (1987). Employee fitness programs: Their impact on the employee and the organization. *Academy of Management Review*, **12**, 511-522.

Faust, H.S., Ferrell, G., Graves, F.W., McDonnell, P., Udow, M., Vermeulen, H., & Weinstock, A. (1983). *Go to health: Final report*. Ann Arbor, MI: Health Analysts.

Gettman, L.R. (1986). Cost/benefit analysis of a corporate fitness program. *Fitness in Business*, **1**(1), 11-17.

Gibbs, J.O., Mulvaney, D., Henes, C., & Reed, R.W. (1985). Work site health promotion: Five-year trend in employee health care costs. *Journal of Occupational Medicine*, **27**, 826-830.

Gladwell, M. (1991, April 23). Health costs' share of GNP up sharply. *The Washington Post*, p. A5.

Golaszewski, T., Lynch, W., Clearie, A., & Vickery, D.M. (1989). The relationship between retrospective health insurance claims and a health risk appraisal-generated measure of health status. *Journal of Occupational Medicine*, **31**, 262-264.

Grana, J. (1985). Weighing the costs and benefits of worksite health promotion. *Corporate Commentary*, **1**(5), 18-19.

Green, L., & Kreuter, M.W. (1991). *Health promotion planning: An educational and environmental approach*. Mountainview, CA: Mayfield.

Herzlinger, R.E., & Schwartz, J. (1985, July/August). How companies tackle health care costs: Part I. *Harvard Business Review*, **63**(4), 69-81.

Hoffman, J.J., Jr., & Hobson, C.J. (1984). Physical fitness and employee effectiveness. *Personnel Administrator*, **29**(4), 101-113, 126.

Hollenback, J., & Heck, S.K. (1991, March). *GE Aircraft Engines Fitness Center cost effectiveness study*. Cincinnati: Office of Wellness Programs, GE Aircraft Engines.

Holzbach, R.L., Piserchia, P.V., McFadden, D.W., Hartwell, T.D., Herrmann, A., & Fielding, J.E. (1990). Effect of a comprehensive health promotion program on employee attitudes. *Journal of Occupational Medicine*, **32**, 973-978.

Horowitz, S.M. (1987). Effects of a worksite wellness program on absenteeism and health care costs in a small federal agency. *Fitness in Business*, **1**(5), 167-172.

Howard, J., & Mikalachki, A. (1979). Fitness and employee productivity. *Canadian Journal of Applied Sport Sciences*, **4**(3), 191-198.

Jacobson, M.I., Yenney, S.L., & Bisgard, J.C. (1990). An organizational perspective on worksite health promotion. *Occupational Medicine: State of the Art Reviews*, **5**, 653-664.

Jones, R.C., Bly, J.L., & Richardson, J.E. (1990). A study of a work site health promotion program and absenteeism. *Journal of Occupational Medicine*, **32**, 95-99.

Jose, W.S., II, Anderson, D.R., & Haight, S.A. (1987). The StayWell strategy for health care cost containment. In J. Opatz (Ed.), *Health promotion evaluation: Measuring the organizational impact* (pp. 15-34). Stevens Point, WI: National Wellness Institute.

Karch, R.C., Newton, D.L., Schaeffer, M.A., Zoltick, J.M., Zajtchuk, R., & Rumbaugh, J.H. (1988). *Cost-benefit and cost-effectiveness measures of health promotion in a military-civilian staff*. Washington, DC: American University, National Center for Health Fitness.

Karch, R.C., Schaeffer, M.A., Stevenson, M.O., Newton, D.L., Krieger, M.J., & Snelling, A.M. (1991). *Effectiveness and benefit measures of the Headquarters, Army Materiel Command health program 1985-1989*. Washington, DC: American University, National Center for Health Fitness.

Katz, P.P., & Showstack, J.A. (1990). Is it worth it? Evaluating the economic impact of worksite health promotion. *Occupational Medicine: State of the Art Reviews*, **5**, 837-850.

Kiefhaber, A., & Goldbeck, W. (1983). An expensive view of worksite wellness. In J.E. Mammer III & B.J. Sox Jacobs (Eds.), *Marketing and managing health care* (pp. 37-54). Memphis: University of Tennessee, Center for the Health Sciences.

Linden, V. (1969). Absence from work and physical fitness. *British Journal of Industrial Medicine*, **26**, 47-53.

Loomis, C.J. (1989, February 27). The killer cost stalking business. *Fortune,* pp. 58-68.

Lynch, W.D., Golaszewski, T.J., Clearie, A.F., Snow, D., & Vickery, D.M. (1990). Impact of a facility-based corporate fitness program on the number of absences from work due to illness. *Journal of Occupational Medicine,* **32**, 9-12.

Muchinsky, P.M. (1977). Employee absenteeism: A review of the literature. *Journal of Vocational Behavior,* **10**, 316-341.

Murphy, R.J., Gasparotto, G., & Opatz, J.P. (1987). Current issues in the evaluation of worksite health promotion programs. In J.P. Opatz (Ed.), *Health promotion evaluation: Measuring the organizational impact* (pp. 1-14). Stevens Point, WI: National Wellness Institute.

O'Donnell, M.P. (1986). Definition of health promotion. *American Journal of Health Promotion,* **1**(1), 4-5.

O'Donnell, M.P. (1988). Cost benefit analysis is not cost effective. *American Journal of Health Promotion,* **3**(1), 74-75.

Office of the Assistant Secretary for Health and the Surgeon General. (1979). *Healthy people: The Surgeon General's report on health promotion and disease prevention* (USDHEW [PHS] Publication No. 79-55071). Washington, DC: U.S. Department of Health, Education, & Welfare.

Patterson, D.C. (1986). Can a company evaluate the costs/benefits of its wellness efforts? *Risk Management,* **33**(11), 30-36.

Pender, N.J., Smith, L.C., & Vernof, J.A. (1987). Building better workers. *American Association of Occupational Health Nursing,* **35**, 386-390.

Reed, R.W. (1985). Health promotion service: Evaluation and impact study. In Barbara B. Minckley (Ed.), *Proceedings of 6th annual meeting, Midwest Alliance in Nursing* (pp. 31-43). Indianapolis: Midwest Alliance in Nursing.

Reed, R.W., Mulvaney, D.E., Billingham, R.E., & Skinner, T.W. (1986). *Health promotion service evaluation and impact study.* Indianapolis: Benchmark Press.

Rhodes, E.C., & Dunwoody, D. (1980). Physiological and attitudinal changes in those involved in an employee fitness program. *Canadian Journal of Public Health,* **71**, 331-336.

Rodnick, J.E. (1982). Health behavior changes associated with health hazard appraisal counseling in an occupational setting. *Preventive Medicine,* **11**, 583-594.

Rudman, W.J. (1987). Do onsite health and fitness programs affect worker productivity? *Fitness in Business,* **2**(1), 2-8.

Shephard, R.J., Corey, P., & Cox, M. (1982a). Health hazard appraisal—the influence of an employee fitness programme. *Canadian Journal of Public Health,* **73**, 183-187.

Shephard, R.J., Corey, P., Renzland, P., & Cox, M. (1982b). The influence of an employee fitness and lifestyle modification program upon medical care costs. *Canadian Journal of Public Health,* **73**, 259-263.

Shephard, R.J., Cox, M., & Corey, P. (1981). Fitness program participation: Its effect on worker performance. *Journal of Occupational Medicine, 23*, 359-363.

Sloan, R.P., Gruman, J.C., & Allegrante, J.P. (1987). *Investing in employee health—A guide to effective health promotion in the workplace.* San Francisco: Jossey-Bass.

Sink, D.S., Tuttle, T.C., & DeVries, S.J. (1984). Productivity measurement and evaluation: What is available? *National Productivity Review, 3*, 265-287.

Smith, K.W., McKinlay, S.M., & Thorington, B.D. (1987). The validity of health risk appraisal instruments for assessing coronary heart disease risk. *American Journal of Public Health, 77*, 419-424.

Spilman, M.A., Goetz, A., Schultz, J., Bellingham, R., & Johnson, D. (1986). Effects of a corporate health promotion program. *Journal of Occupational Medicine, 28*, 285-290.

Terborg, J.R. (1986). Health promotion at the worksite: A research challenge for personnel and human resources management. In K.M. Rowland & G.R. Ferris (Eds.), *Research in personnel and human resources management, 4*, pp. 225-267. Greenwich, CT: JAI Press.

Tucker, L.A., Aldana, S.G., & Friedman, G.M. (1990). Cardiovascular fitness and absenteeism in 8,301 employed adults. *American Journal of Health Promotion, 5*(2), 140-145.

United States Bureau of the Census. (1990). National health expenditures: 1970 to 1987. *Statistical abstract of the United States: 1990* (110th edition). Washington, DC.

Van Tuinen, M., & Land, G. (1986). Smoking and excess sick leave in a department of health. *Journal of Occupational Medicine, 28*, 33-35.

Wagner, E.H., Beery, W.L., Schoenbach, V.J., & Graham, R.M. (1982). An assessment of health hazard/health risk appraisal. *American Journal of Public Health, 72*, 347-351.

Warner, K.E., Wickizer, T.M., Wolfe, R.A., Schildroth, J.E., & Samuelson, M.H. (1988). Economic implications of workplace health promotion programs: Review of the literature. *Journal of Occupational Medicine, 30*, 106-112.

Wood, E.A., Olmstead, G.W., & Craig, J.L. (1989). An evaluation of lifestyle risk factors and absenteeism after two years in a worksite health promotion program. *American Journal of Health Promotion, 4*(2), 128-133.

Yarvote, P.M., McDonagh, T.J., Goldman, M.E., & Zuckerman, J. (1974). Organization and evaluation of a physical fitness program in industry. *Journal of Occupational Medicine, 16*, 589-598.

Yen, L.T., Edington, D.W., & Witting, P. (1991). Associations between health risk appraisal scores and employee medical claims costs in a manufacturing company. *American Journal of Health Promotion, 6*(1), 46-54.

Chapter 5

Evaluation:
Guidelines for the Accountable
Health Promotion Professional

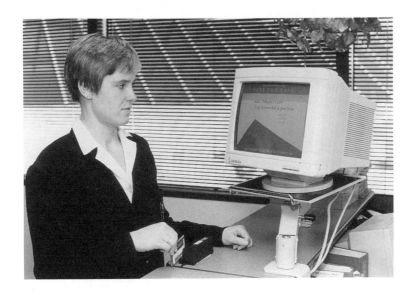

Steve Hoover
Marilyn Jensen
Robert Murphy
David Anderson

Sally, a health promotion professional in a midwestern corporation, is
asked to defend her worksite health promotion program for reducing stress

among employees. She "knows" it has been effective; she is aware of employees who have sought help and expressed their appreciation for learning strategies to reduce stress and increase their productivity. The chief executive officer has asked for data regarding the effectiveness of the program and justification for its cost.

Jane has been hired to develop a smoking cessation program for employees in a large manufacturing company, but from her initial discussions, Jane sees that there is considerable resistance from some managers to funding such activities. Where should she begin?

Jerry, a health promotion professional who has developed a weight loss program and stress management course for his company's employees, has collected data regarding the program, but the data show no change. Jerry believes the program has had impact, but he has no idea how to document its effectiveness. These data are important to support his request for expansion of the health promotion program to include other lifestyle risk factors.

A company president must make some decisions on cutting expenditures; she comes to you for data regarding your worksite health promotion program and a cost analysis. Can you justify continuation of the program and your position?

Health promotion programs at the worksite have increased dramatically in recent years. As health care professionals and organization managers have recognized the needs and benefits of worksite health promotion, programs to improve the health and lifestyles of the work force have proliferated. At the same time has come concern for the effectiveness of various health promotion approaches. Increasingly, decision-makers are looking for evidence regarding the costs and benefits of all programs, including worksite health promotion offerings. Inherent in this concern for accountability is the desire to have some measures of outcomes that can be used to provide future direction; principles of program evaluation can play a role in this regard. As is indicated by the opening scenarios, there are many faces to program evaluation; this chapter will follow Jane through her situation to illustrate the text.

Traditionally, program evaluation has been considered after the fact, leaving program implementers to scramble when required to provide data on the effectiveness of their programs. However, there is a growing realization that a well-designed, dynamic evaluation is an integral component of a comprehensive decision-making strategy. Managers are thus increasingly concerned with identifying early in program development the issues or outcomes that will provide appropriate data for ongoing, informed decisions.

In this chapter we provide health promotion professionals with basic concepts regarding the evaluation of worksite health promotion programs with the goal of seeking information by which appropriate decisions may be made. Because organizational decisions often differ depending on the stage of program implementation, and because different evaluation designs or strategies can be used depending on the nature of the decisions to be made, we will present several evaluation models and discuss their strengths and weaknesses.

As in any decision-making process, the key to success is planning. There are specific steps to follow in planning an evaluation:

1. Identify the major stakeholders in the evaluation.
2. Establish the criteria and time lines for program outcomes.
3. Identify sources of evaluation data.
4. Select models or designs that address the questions to be asked.
5. Identify, or create, the data collection instruments and procedures.
6. Plan effective times for collecting data.
7. Select data analyses appropriate to the questions asked and the nature of the data.
8. Develop an effective format for communicating evaluation results so that they will be used effectively.
9. Develop a process for implementing recommendations.

Identify the Major Stakeholders

Those planning an evaluation need to be certain that they get adequate input from the people who will use the data to make decisions. These stakeholders need to be a part of the evaluation's initial design. Otherwise evaluators run the risk of gathering insufficient or inappropriate data.

For example, even though self-report has been shown to be a valid measure of smoking status (Petitti, Friedman, & Kahn, 1981), it may be advisable to evaluate using a more costly biometric screen if key stakeholders are skeptical about self-report measures. Taking the time to explore with stakeholders their concerns and their desires for particular information clarifies the nature of the evaluation and ensures collecting data they will support as valid.

As the first step in evaluation, Jane proceeds to identify the major stake-holders in the decision-making process to develop a company smoking cessation program. The president of the firm, a long-time heavy smoker who has recently had a heart attack, is the prime supporter for expending funds for a smoking cessation program. Jane learns in discussions with managers that some of them are concerned about the relationship between smoking and health care claims and sick leave requests. However, many are skeptical about the benefits of health promotion programs. Are there others resistant to the plan? Who will be involved in the decision-making process and program implementation? What role will employees and potential program participants play? Jane sets up a series of meetings with managers and employees who will be affected by the program to allow their input into program development and evaluation and to set the stage for ongoing communication about the effectiveness of the program.

Establish Criteria for Program Outcomes

To be most effective, program evaluation should be a dynamic process integrally linked to the organization's decision-making process. As the company's needs change, the evaluation must also change. Table 5.1 presents a model for conceptualizing the role of program evaluation within the context of a decision-making process.

Table 5.1 identifies three stages of program development, a set of corresponding questions, and potential evaluation designs that could be used to address these questions. After the stakeholders are identified, efforts should be directed toward establishing the evaluation questions and program outcomes that will be the criteria by which the program's effectiveness will be judged. As indicated in Table 5.1, the specific questions will vary depending on the existing program.

Related to the planning of program evaluations is the issue of goals versus objectives. Stakeholders often have in mind only broad goals such as increasing worker productivity or morale. However, these are too broad to be measured. Evaluation planning must turn these broad goal statements into clear objectives that can be directly measured. For instance, though the goals may be increased productivity and improved employee morale, specific objectives might be to reduce absenteeism due to illness by 10% in 3 years and to increase employee satisfaction with the company's support for good health from 10% to 60% within 1 year.

Not only is it necessary to work closely with stakeholders in establishing the outcomes, it is also vital to establish a time frame for conducting the evaluation. In most cases decision-makers need information in a timely manner. Data that come in *after* the decisions are made will be useless and will reflect poorly on both the program and the evaluator. Companies tend to make decisions on annual cycles; therefore, design your evaluation (e.g., an organization-wide risk profile) to provide up-to-date results before decisions are made about funding.

Table 5.1
Model for Conceptualizing the Role of Program Evaluation
in the Decision-Making Process

Stages in program development	Types of data needed/questions	Relevant evaluation models/designs
Program development and design	Why is the program needed? Who would benefit from the program? What are the options available? What are the costs involved? What are the expected outcomes? What form should the program take?	Needs assessment Pilot program
Program implementation	Is the program being implemented as planned? Are resources being used as intended? Are there changes in the design or delivery of the program that should be made? Are staff adequately trained? Are the "right" people being served?	Formative evaluation Fiscal evaluation Goal-free evaluation
Program assessment and effectiveness	Were the intended outcomes achieved? What benefits have accrued because of the program? Are the changes significant? What are the economic benefits from the program? What additional, nonplanned effects occurred?	Experimental and quasi-experimental designs Goal-based evaluation Cost-benefit evaluation Goal-free evaluation

To facilitate discussion about the need for a smoking cessation program, Jane scheduled meetings with stakeholders to ask the program development questions in Table 5.1. Although Jane saw the company's need for a comprehensive health promotion program, she recognized that an effective smoking cessation program could be an important first step in the process. Jane learned from the discussions that the president was highly motivated to reduce employee smoking, and some managers expressed concern about the health risks associated with the high rate of employee smoking. However, she needed to translate these general goals and concerns into specific objectives with criteria that would determine if they had been accomplished and time lines for completion. After several meetings with the stakeholders, Jane established these objectives:

1. Conduct a needs assessment.
   - By February, complete health risk assessments of all employees to assess smoking and other health risk behaviors, and collect and summarize paid sick leave records and absenteeism data to establish a baseline.
   - By March, survey employees regarding their interest in smoking cessation and the kind of program they would find most helpful.
2. Develop a pilot program.
   - By March, review the literature regarding the most effective smoking cessation strategies and worksite health promotion programs.
   - By April, identify expected process and outcome measures by which the effectiveness of the program will be evaluated; complete an evaluation design; and identify program participants and collect baseline data on their smoking habits.
3. Implement the pilot program.

After reviewing the literature on smoking cessation programs at the worksite, Jane decided that programs developed by Glasgow et al. (1991), Bertera, Oehl, and Telepchak (1990), and Wood, Olmstead, and Craig (1989) seemed applicable to her worksite and potentially effective in addressing her company's needs for a smoking program. The focus of intervention would be monthly incentives for reductions in smoking by program participants based on self-report and biochemical verification.

After discussions with the major stakeholders, Jane established these process and outcome measures:

Process measures

a. Data will be collected regarding participation rates.

b. Data will be collected regarding the implementation of the program (review of program records).

Outcome measures

a. By the end of the program year, at least 25% of program participants will be abstaining from smoking as determined by self-report and carbon monoxide readings.

b. Smoking abstinence rates will be maintained through a 6-month follow-up.

c. Participants will demonstrate an increased knowledge regarding risks of smoking.

d. Absenteeism due to illness will decrease by 25% among participants.

Identify Sources of Evaluation Data

When establishing the outcomes for the program, you must also locate appropriate sources from which the data will be collected. Posavac and Carey (1992) recommend six potential sources of evaluation data: program records; program participants; program staff; significant others; evaluator observations; and community indexes.

Program records represent the data sources that are the most manageable, because they do not involve going beyond records that are routinely collected regarding a program's operations. Specifically, these data sources include company records such as absenteeism reports, medical and health care claims, workers' compensation claims, disability claims, life insurance claims, sick leave usage and payment, and performance appraisals.

A major limitation of program records is the limited breadth of information. Unless planned early, the records may not contain the information needed to answer specific questions. Another limitation lies in the use of health care claims to measure program effects. Several authors have identified the problems associated with using such claims records (Lynch, Teitelbaum, & Main, 1991a, 1991b). Anderson and Jose (1987) point out that

a very large data base, although often not available to researchers in this field, is essential in most analyses involving health care claim data for several reasons. First, the distribution of typical claim indicators, such as annual claims per employee, includes many employees with no claim costs and others with claim costs 10 to 100 or more times the mean. Such skewed distributions result in standard deviations often exceeding twice the group mean. Second, base rates for other important indicators such as those for hospital admissions or cardiovascular disease are relatively low. Finally, statistical "outliers" like very high claim costs are often related to the predictor variables being tested (e.g., hypertension) and ideally should not be removed from analyses designed to specify the effects of these predictors.

Thus, while preliminary trends linking lifestyle risks to health care claim costs were noted in StayWell evaluation reports as early as 1983, practical applications were not recommended until results could be replicated on a larger, more reliable data set. (p. 88)

Thus, due to the skewed nature of health care claim data, the large variations in the data, the time lag in effects having a visible influence on claim data, and the contamination of claim data by other variables, the authors of this chapter urge caution when using this form of program record: The evaluator must be aware of these limitations and well versed in appropriate statistical analyses (e.g., loglinear modeling).

A major source of data in any evaluation will be those for whom the program is intended. Program participants serve as subjects for questionnaires, interviews, physiological and psychological assessments, and attitudinal studies. Participants are in the unique position of being able to comment directly on the impact of the program. Program evaluators, however, need to be cautious when using information from participants, because there may be some confusion between participants' perception of program effects and actual behavioral changes. Employees may be able to tell an evaluator how much they like or dislike specific program activities; however, they are a much less reliable source for assessment of design features that require expertise, for example, behavior modification methods and outcomes. Therefore, evaluators must define measures appropriate to the desired changes in behavior, not only in how participants perceive them, but also designing or selecting procedures and instruments that will assess actual changes.

Program staff can also provide information on the operations of the program, costs, time involvement, and numerous other aspects, because of their unique perspective. Data from program staff is valuable information, because staff have ample opportunity to provide feedback on how the program actually operates. In cases where evaluations looked only at the outcomes when concluding whether programs were effective, none of the data collected addressed why the programs succeeded or failed. However, unless program staff view the evaluation process as means by which to improve program operations, they may be reluctant to make any other comments than positive ones.

Program staff can also be an excellent source of qualitative data. Anecdotal feedback or monthly activity reports by program staff can be rich sources of process or formative evaluation data. This information can aid in decisions about how the programs are delivered to clients. Such qualitative data provide a contrast to the more traditional, hard data characteristic of research designs.

Depending on the questions to be answered, data may have to be collected from those who are not in the program itself, but who are directly affected by changes in program participants. Significant others include spouses, children, relatives, coworkers, and supervisors who may be able to observe individuals in settings other than the worksite. For example, Jose and Anderson (1991) cite evidence from coworkers who did not participate in program activities that those who did participate showed improved health habits. Spouses can serve as valuable sources regarding the extent to which their husbands or wives maintain healthy lifestyles away from the worksite and how changes in health habits affect the employed partners' lives generally.

In some cases it is most effective for the evaluator to personally collect observational data on program operations. This could be done either through a naturalistic or ethnographic study or by having independent observers monitor specific aspects of a program. Because evaluators often have a stake in the success of the programs (e.g., their continued employment), asking one or more independent observers to look carefully at the program's operations may be more desirable. This would be particularly useful if their results were communicated directly to the stakeholders to corroborate the information and conclusions drawn by the in-house evaluator.

Finally, consider effects of the program as a whole. Posavac and Carey (1992) suggest looking at community-level indexes as a source of data; but it would also be reasonable to review organization-level indexes, such as absenteeism, health care costs, or productivity data, to see the extent to which a company's health promotion programs are having an impact.

Jose and Anderson (1991) developed a model that shows the impact of program components on both employee and employer benefits (see Figure 5.1). Developing such a model allows program planners and evaluators to track the impact of their health promotion offerings, to establish outcomes, and to access appropriate sources of data.

To facilitate the process of designing an evaluation after the first two steps have been concluded, we created a matrix that allows the evaluator to "see" the various elements of the evaluation and how these elements support one another. Figure 5.2 presents this evaluation planning matrix. The components across the top of the matrix represent the outcomes or criteria that have been established to define program effectiveness. Sources of data are listed along the vertical axis of the matrix. The cells of the matrix represent planning areas wherein the evaluator can make decisions regarding data collection from the corresponding sources, what form that data will take (e.g., observations, pre- and postassessments, interviews, etc.), and when the data are to be collected. Once completed, the matrix serves as a master plan for the evaluation and can be shared with stakeholders to ensure that it will in fact generate data appropriate to their needs.

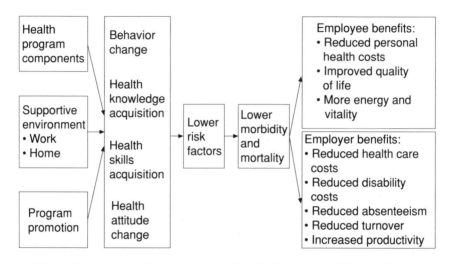

Figure 5.1 The StayWell process model. *Note.* From "Control Data's StayWell Program: A Health Cost Management Strategy" by W.S. Jose and D.R. Anderson. In *Perspectives in Behavioral Medicine: Health at Work* (pp. 49-72) by S.M. Weiss, J.E. Fielding, and A. Baum (Eds.), 1991, Hillsdale, NJ: Lawrence Erlbaum Associates. Reprinted by permission.

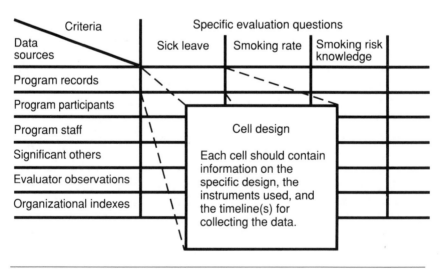

Figure 5.2 Program evaluation planning matrix.

Select Evaluation Models or Designs

Initially, most program evaluations were designed to establish a cause-and-effect relationship between the program and the outcomes and used a traditional social science model or true experiment. However, because of the nature of worksite health promotion programs, there are several potential threats to internal validity (e.g., selection, mortality, etc.), which often militate against the use of a true experimental design. (For a complete list, see Conrad, Conrad, & Walcott-McQuigg, 1991.)

A major limitation of true experimental design is the long-term nature of programs and their results or outcomes, which make it virtually impossible to "sell" such designs to management. Furthermore, even if management were willing to accept it, truly experimental design can be implemented only in very narrow areas, because of restrictions regarding random assignment and problems associated with "denying" treatment to qualified employees.

In lieu of the more traditional, true experimental designs, a number of evaluation models have been proposed that, although not as straightforward regarding cause and effect, can be used in combinations to evince overall program effectiveness. Jose, Anderson, and Haight (1987) pointed out that by utilizing a combination of designs that have different threats to internal validity, the evaluator can begin to establish a *pattern* of results that address program effectiveness. Nonexperimental models of evaluation include pre- or nonexperimental and quasi-experimental designs, formative or process evaluation, goal-based evaluation, goal-free evaluation, single-case designs, and cost-benefit or cost-effectiveness analysis.

Pre- or Nonexperimental Designs

Cook and Campbell (1979) identified three designs that do not allow the determination of causative relations between treatment and outcome. One such design is the posttest-only design in which observations, tests, and questionnaires are administered to participants after the program. Surveying employees on their degree of satisfaction is an example of this type of design. Though the results may provide some indication of general satisfaction with the program, there is no way to assess real behavioral changes because there are no comparisons made between the participants' post- and preexisting conditions (posttest/pretest) or between participants' and nonparticipants' conditions.

A second preexperimental design includes a set of posttest-only observations of a nonequivalent control group that does not receive the program treatments. This is a fairly common practice when programs have been established before considering how to evaluate their effectiveness. In this case, an evaluator must attempt to locate individuals who are similar to those receiving the treatment and compare their conditions using the outcome measures. Though this design might provide more information than the single-group, posttest-only design, it still does not allow an evaluator to state with certainty that the treatment is effective. This design can be more useful if the evaluator can collect preexisting data, which can serve as pretest data, from company records. Though this cannot replace better-planned evaluations, tentative data can be salvaged, which might be helpful in future program development.

A third form of common preexperimental design assesses only program participants before and after the treatment. The most obvious flaw in this design is the inability to attribute changes in participants to the program itself. Alternative factors could contribute to the observed changes. Alternative factors are those not directly manipulated in the study, but correlated with the outcome measures. These could include any number of factors, such as preexisting differences, history effects, or differing motivational characteristics. Although it is impossible to make direct causal relationships, it is possible to determine whether any changes occurred and the extent of those changes. For example, if Jane's smoking cessation program shows no change in program participants from pretest to posttest, then it could reasonably be assumed that the program is ineffective and needs modification. Furthermore, if participants in Jane's program reduce their smoking to the desired levels from pretest to posttest, then, from the point of view of the participants and the sponsoring employer, the program could be considered a success. This does not mean that this type of design is as appropriate as quasi-experimental designs, only that in some instances no other type of design may be possible. This situation could occur when the program is designed for all employees because management chooses not to "exclude" any eligible employees, as would be the case with a true experimental design.

Quasi-Experimental Designs

Cook and Campbell (1979) present a number of designs that allow for some degree of causal interpretation. In essence, these designs do so by either increasing the number of observations of a single group (see "Single-Case Designs," p. 112) or including a control group, which does not receive the program. They also include designs that incorporate both the control group and the number of observations. As mentioned previously, the designs increase in their ability to establish causal relationships between changes and treatment as far as such comparisons can be made. These comparisons are limited because individuals are seldom randomly assigned to treatment or control groups. Usually, employees are invited to participate in a company's health promotion offerings, and when individuals have self-selected to participate, questions arise regarding whether the treatment, the nature of those who self-selected, or a combination of these two factors caused any changes observed in the participants. Nonetheless, pre- and postassessment with nonequivalent control groups is a very common design and may be the best option open to an evaluator. In this case, the evaluator may wish to design a series of replications to identify possible program effects (Jose et al., 1987).

Another alternative when the evaluator is faced with a design such as the pre- and posttest nonequivalent control group is to make statistical adjustments using preexisting differences between groups. One such procedure uses analysis of covariance (ANCOVA), in which mean differences between the control and experimental groups are tested for significance after the means have been "adjusted" based on preexisting conditions that are related to the outcome measures. Though this may provide some evidence of program effects, it is limited it at least two ways. First, the procedure requires that the evaluator identify variables that are related to the outcome measures (e.g., age, sex, and education). This can be done by looking at correlations between preexisting variables and outcomes, but it is not possible to identify *all* possible related variables. Second, the ANCOVA procedure tends to underadjust for initial differences; therefore, truly program-caused effects may not be identified.

Formative, or Process, Evaluation

Whereas other designs are intended to look specifically at the outcomes (i.e., effects) of the program, formative, or process, evaluation is designed to assess the extent to which the program treatments are being implemented as planned. This evaluation design is often more qualitative than others with its greater emphasis on use of questionnaires, interviews, and observations to determine how the program is being implemented, its strengths and weaknesses, and how it might be made more effective.

Formative evaluation is important for making in-progress revisions, but also in more controlled, true or quasi-experimental designs, for the fidelity of the program operations. It is not enough simply to pretest participants and then assess them at the program's end. It is also necessary to look carefully at how individuals are participating to be certain that the program is operating as planned. For example, Jane should ensure that the smoking cessation program is, in fact, being implemented as intended by looking at participation rates, interviewing participants, and having discussions with program staff. Such feedback will reveal the extent to which the program is being delivered in the manner planned to those who should be receiving it.

Goal-Based Versus Goal-Free Evaluation

Much of the discussion so far refers to assessing actual outcomes based upon the planned, or desired outcomes of a program—the objectives or goals for the program. Assessing these outcomes is important in establishing the effectiveness of the program. However, programs can have effects beyond those intended. Jose et al. (1987) point out that among important outcomes of worksite health promotion programs are the changes that occur in people's perceptions of their and others' health-related behaviors and the effects that programs have on the worksite environment. Because these changes may not have been planned or even anticipated, they would have been missed by an assessment directed only toward the program's defined goals.

Unplanned positive and negative side effects of programs should also be included in a complete evaluation. To gather evidence of the program's effectiveness beyond the stated goals, the evaluator must rely on qualitative assessments such as open-ended interviews or questionnaires, observations, and discussions designed to reveal *any* changes. Once observed, these unplanned effects can be included in future planning and evaluation.

Single-Case Designs

Kazdin (1978) and Barlow and Hersen (1981) state that the rationale of single-case designs is similar to that of traditional group research. The essence of group research, as well as single-case research, is comparison of performance under different conditions. How the comparison is made, though, differs in each situation. In traditional research, different groups of individuals (or in some instances, the same group) are exposed to different conditions. Single-case designs typically observe an individual's behavior for a period before one or more conditions are changed. Data collected from a subject under differing conditions provide information about present performance, predict the level of future performance, and test the accuracy of earlier predictions. The successive changes in conditions provide opportunities to collect information analogous to that obtained through traditional research, which compares the performances of experimental and control groups. When information is collected this way, observed changes in individual performance can be more confidently attributed to specific interventions rather than to events that parallel them but are unrelated.

There are many types of single-case designs from which an evaluator may choose depending on the circumstances and objectives of the specific evaluation project. Barlow and Hersen (1981) list and extensively discuss the procedures, strengths, and limitations of many of them. We will restrict our discussion to multiple baseline designs. These are single-case designs that are particularly well adapted to assessing the effects of health promotion interventions, given the practical demands of operating in a typical work setting. They are not only applicable across the widest range of evaluation conditions but also can be quickly learned, readily accepted, and easily implemented by direct service staff (Nietzel, Winett, MacDonald, & Davidson, 1977).

Multiple baseline designs provide evidence that a particular intervention produces an effect by showing that behavior change occurs if, and only if, the intervention is present. One of three types of multiple baselines can be used whenever the situation calls for data collection (a) across a variety of behaviors of the same individual or group within a given setting, (b) across a variety of settings for the same behavior of an individual or group, or (c) across a variety of individuals or groups displaying the same behavior in the same setting. Technically, only two behaviors, individual groups, or settings are needed to show intervention-produced effects, but several investigators suggest that in most cases three or four replications are necessary to provide a convincing demonstration (Barlow & Hersen, 1981).

There are strengths and weaknesses to each evaluation design, and the evaluator needs first to look carefully at the questions to be addressed by the evaluation and then choose the design or designs that will provide the most useful information for those decision-makers.

To assess the effectiveness of the smoking cessation program, Jane chose a multiple baseline design. To establish the impact of the incentive-based program on rate of smoking, Jane identified three groups of employees (i.e., employees in three sales divisions of the company). She asked volunteers from the three groups to complete questionnaires regarding their smoking behavior and to submit to carbon monoxide tests at the beginning of the program. Next, she implemented the program first for one group and then at 6-month intervals for the remaining two groups, each time collecting data to provide an ongoing baseline of smoking behavior. She also collected data regarding process measures on a regular basis to ensure the adequacy of program implementation and to make changes where necessary. Both before and after the intervention, she collected data regarding outcome measures (e.g., smoking and absenteeism).

Thus, Jane was able to evaluate the effectiveness of the smoking cessation program by comparing data before and after intervention for three different groups of individuals who had entered the program at staggered intervals. By using this evaluation design, Jane was able to make conclusions regarding the program's impact and to make comparisons without denying the intervention to interested employees.

Cost-Benefit and Cost-Effectiveness Analysis

Similarly to other programs, worksite health promotion programs can have costs without benefits, but they cannot have benefits without costs.

Therefore, ever increasing numbers of health promotion directors and coordinators are being required to discuss with corporate decision-makers not only who they are and what they do, but how much they cost. This has heightened interest among program evaluators in various cost evaluation techniques, ranging from purely descriptive procedures, such as cost analysis and cost outcome analysis, to those that directly compare program costs to program benefits, such as output value analysis and cost-benefit analysis.

Although there are many cost evaluation procedures, two that have received the most attention among health care professionals are cost-benefit and cost-effectiveness analysis. Because both procedures will probably become even more prevalent in the future, it is extremely important that their correct use, as well as their limitations, be well understood (Murphy, Gasparotto, & Opatz, 1987).

According to Opatz, Chenoweth, and Kaman (1991), cost-benefit analysis involves assigning a dollar value to all of the costs associated with implementing a health promotion program and to all the benefits that result. Though there are several ways of numerically presenting the result of such analyses, the most common method is a simple ratio of benefit to cost. Any result greater than 1 indicates a net profit and any result less than 1 a net loss.

Cost-effectiveness analysis involves determining the dollar costs of implementing the program and then, rather than calculating the financial benefits, measuring them in nonmonetary units such as increased years of life, reduction in risk factor status, and improved quality of life. This procedure is most often used to rank various program alternatives according to the size of their effect relative to their costs.

Several investigators (Banta & Luce, 1983; Jones & Baker, 1986; Murphy, Elias, Gasparotto, & Huset, 1987; Thompson, 1980) provide excellent descriptions and illustrations of these analytic techniques applied to health promotion activities.

Identify Data Collection Instruments and Procedures

A major concern of evaluation is the reliability and validity of the instruments and procedures used to obtain data. A full treatment of issues surrounding instrumentation are beyond the scope of this chapter, but you should try to determine how reliable and valid the instruments used to collect data are for the sample population. Evaluators often create their own instruments to assess program effects, particularly where attitudes and perceptions of program effects are considered.

You must be cautious regarding the use of instruments that have not been psychometrically analyzed. Though reliability of assessment is crucial, the validity of the instruments used to gather the data is of greater concern. Instruments may seem appropriate for the intended purposes of the evaluation, however, "face" validity does not ensure that data from the instrument will, in fact, prove valid or provide information necessary to make informed decisions.

If at all possible, use existing instruments that have shown some degree of reliability and validity. If you use instruments of your own design, provide some evidence of the reliability and validity of those instruments and procedures. This information should be included in the final report under "limitations" of the evaluation, and you should assess the impact on the program's results.

Plan Data Collection

There are several factors to consider when planning the collection of data during an evaluation. First, through discussions with the stakeholders, determine when the results of the evaluation are needed for decision making. Though these decisions are generally made on a fiscal year basis, you must budget your time for getting the instruments coded and analyzed, the results compiled, and conclusions drawn. Working backward from the due date of the final report and allocating time for delay in participants' response to questionnaires or for conducting a follow-up survey will help you complete the study on time.

A second issue that should be considered when planning data collection has to do with the timing of events and data collection. Depending on when questionnaires are administered, employee attitudes may be different than those during other times of the year. Assessing attitudes toward eating and exercise immediately after Thanksgiving may yield different results than doing so in the spring when people are concerned about summer and the beach.

Finally, placing test dates on the planning matrix in Figure 5.2 and sharing this with supervisors and stakeholders will help ensure that the data will be collected on time and that special events will have been identified in advance.

Select Data Analysis Procedures

Which procedures you use to analyze data depend on the nature of the data, how it was collected, and the questions to be answered. Code qualitative data from interviews, questionnaires, and observations first into categories that are either predetermined or suggested by the data itself. Then look for information from trends in participant or staff comments and observations and for evidence of unplanned program effects, which are particularly relevant to qualitative or goal-free evaluations.

Data from instruments chosen to identify changes related to program effects usually require statistical analysis, and you must consider the probability of the results being due to chance rather than to the program. Give careful consideration *before* the data are collected to the types of questions to be answered. In most cases, you are interested in pretest-to-posttest changes, comparing mean responses between groups, and the extent to which variables are interrelated. In some cases, you may be interested in the characteristics of a particular group of individuals, for example, the risk factor profiles of those who have high health care-related costs compared to those who have lower costs. A full treatment of matching analysis procedures to the data and questions to be answered is beyond the scope of this chapter; you can find excellent decision trees for assisting in analysis in Saslow (1982), Bausell (1986), and Linton and Gallo (1975). More sophisticated analyses, such as analysis of covariance and discriminant analysis, can be found in Johnson and Wichern (1988), Tabachnick and Fidell (1989), and Diekhoff (1992).

Communicate Results

Once the data are "in," you must effectively communicate the results of the evaluation to those who need the information to make decisions. Writing and presenting the results are important steps in "selling" the results of your evaluation and its recommendations. Though your full report should include the questions that were considered, the design of the evaluation, how the data were analyzed, conclusions, recommendations, and limitations, it is often appropriate to provide an executive summary. This is particularly true for decision-makers who want clear, concise information. The executive summary should provide a brief overview of the study, the results, and recommendations for future programming options. If some wish to review the complete study, they can read the full report later.

A major focus of the stakeholders will be the effectiveness of the program and what changes should be implemented in the future, including cost projections derived from needs revealed by the evaluation. Overly broad generalizations should be avoided. Tie each recommendation to specific results indicated by the study so that stakeholders can see directly the logic behind your recommendations.

Implement Recommendations

Much time and effort goes into the planning and implementing of an evaluation project, but the process does not end with the presentation of your results and recommendations. For the evaluation to be truly effective, you must include a plan for implementing the recommendations. If key stakeholders were involved in the initial planning, implementation should be easy to get started. However, if these key stakeholders were not involved, they may have less interest in acting on the recommendations.

Implementation requires meeting with stakeholders to establish time lines and cost projections for putting recommendations into practice. One effective approach is to take a recommendation and determine what can be done in the short run (e.g., the first year), and what should be planned for over the long run (e.g., a 5-year plan). Be very specific when making these plans. At a minimum, each recommendation should have a set of specific outcomes or objectives, a time line for implementation, and a schedule of projected costs and should designate who is responsible. When well organized, such plans can help a future evaluation process establish whether these recommendations have been implemented and whether they were effective.

Jane scheduled a series of ongoing meetings with stakeholders to apprise them of the status of program implementation and to identify changes that resulted from the formative evaluation. On the basis of her evaluation, Jane recommended expansion of the smoking cessation program to other company divisions. Evaluation data, outcome measures, and the cost-benefit analysis were also important in decision making by stakeholders on including other lifestyle risk factors in future worksite health promotion programs.

Summary

This chapter has discussed several effective evaluation designs for worksite health promotion programs. A process model designed to provide data to be used in making informed decisions has been the basis. Health promotion professionals interested in conducting an evaluation of a worksite health program should use this chapter as a model. Further assistance in planning an evaluation can be found in the *American Journal of Health Promotion* and publications such as the Program Evaluation Series, published by Sage. The Program Evaluation Kit (Morris, 1987) includes basic evaluation designs, procedures for establishing goals and objectives, methods for measuring variables of interest, suggestions for constructing instruments, and data analysis techniques.

Effective evaluations are important to health promotion professionals, assisting them in providing valid, reliable data to decision-makers, continuing and expanding health promotion programs at the worksite, and gauging the benefits to their companies of improved lifestyle and employee health. Health promotion professionals must become more effective in evaluating their offerings, and this chapter should help.

References

Anderson, D.R., & Jose, W.S. (1987). Employee lifestyle and the bottom line: Results from the StayWell evaluation. *Fitness in Business*, **1**(6), 86-91.

Banta, H.D., & Luce, B.R. (1983). Assessing the cost-effectiveness of prevention. *Journal of Community Health*, **8**(3), 145-165.

Barlow, D.H., & Hersen, M. (1981). *Single-case experimental designs: Strategies for studying behavior change* (2nd ed.). New York: Pergamon Press.

Bausell, R. (1986). *A practical guide to conducting empirical research.* New York: Harper & Row.

Bertera, R., Oehl, L., & Telepchak, J. (1990). Self-help versus group approaches to smoking cessation in the workplace: Eighteen-month follow-up cost analysis. *American Journal of Health Promotion*, **4**(3), 187-192.

Conrad, K.M., Conrad, K.J., & Walcott-McQuigg, J. (1991). Threats to internal validity in worksite health promotion program research: Common problems and possible solutions. *American Journal of Health Promotion*, **6**(2), 112-122.

Cook, T.D., & Campbell, D.T. (1979). *Quasi-experimentation: Design and analysis issues for field settings.* Boston: Houghton Mifflin.

Diekhoff, G. (1992). *Statistics for the social and behavioral sciences: Univariate, bivariate, and multivariate.* Dubuque, IA: Brown.

Glasgow, R., Hollis, J., Pettigrew, L., Foster, L., Givi, M., & Morrisette, G. (1991). Implementing a year-long worksite-based incentive program for smoking cessation. *American Journal of Health Promotion*, **5**(3), 192-199.

Johnson, R.A., & Wichern, D.W. (1988). *Applied multivariate statistical analysis* (2nd ed.). Englewood Cliffs, NJ: Prentice Hall.

Jones, L., & Baker, M.R. (1986). The application of health economics to health promotion. *Community Medicine*, **8**(3), 224-229.

Jose, W.S., & Anderson, D.R. (1991). Control Data's StayWell Program: A health cost management strategy. In S.M. Weiss, J. E. Fielding, & A. Baum (Eds.), *Health at work* (pp. 49-72). Hillsdale, NJ: Erlbaum.

Jose, W.S., Anderson, D.R., & Haight, S.A. (1987). The StayWell strategy for health care cost containment. In J. Opatz (Ed.), *Health promotion evaluation: Measuring the organizational impact* (pp. 15-34). Stevens Point, WI: National Wellness Institute.

Kazdin, A. (1978). Methodological and interpretive problems of single-case experimental designs. *Journal of Consulting and Clinical Psychology*, **46**, 629-642.

Linton, M., & Gallo, P. (1975). *The practical statistician: Simplified handbook of statistics*. Monterey, CA: Brooks/Cole.

Lynch, W.D., Teitelbaum, H.S., & Main, D.S. (1991a). The inadequacy of using means to compare medical costs of smokers and nonsmokers. *American Journal of Health Promotion*, **6**(2), 123-128.

Lynch, W.D., Teitelbaum, H.S., & Main, D.S. (1991b). Comparing medical costs by analyzing high-cost cases. *American Journal of Health Promotion*, **6**(3), 206-213.

Morris, L.L. (1987). *Program evaluation kit* (2nd ed.). Newbury Park, CA: Sage.

Murphy, R., Gasparotto, G., & Opatz, J. (1987). Current issues in the evaluation of worksite health promotion programs. In J. Opatz (Ed.), *Health promotion evaluation: Measuring the organizational impact* (pp. 1-14). Stevens Point, WI: National Wellness Institute.

Murphy, R.J., Elias, W.S., Gasparotto, G., & Huset, R.A. (1987). Cost-benefit analysis in worksite health promotion evaluation. *Fitness in Business*, **1**(5), 15-19.

Nietzel, M., Winett, R., MacDonald, M., & Davidson, W. (1977). *Behavioral approaches to community psychology*. New York: Pergamon Press.

Opatz, J., Chenoweth, D., & Kaman, R. (1991, August). *Economic impact of worksite health promotion*. (Available from Association for Worksite Health Promotion, 310 North Alabama Street, Suite A100, Indianapolis, IN 46204).

Petitti, D.B., Friedman, G.D., & Kahn, W. (1981). Accuracy of information on smoking habits provided on self-administered research questionnaires. *American Journal of Public Health*, **71**(3), 308-311.

Posavac, E. J., & Carey, R.G. (1992). *Program evaluation: Methods and case studies* (4th ed.). Englewood Cliffs, NJ: Prentice Hall.

Saslow, C.A. (1982). *Basic research methods*. New York: Random House.

Tabachnick, B., & Fidell, L. (1989). *Using multivariate statistics*. New York: Harper Collins.

Thompson, M. (1980). *Benefit-cost analysis for program evaluation*. Beverly Hills, CA: Sage.

Wood, E., Olmstead, G., & Craig, J. (1989). An evaluation of lifestyle risk factors and absenteeism after two years in a worksite health promotion program. *American Journal of Health Promotion*, **4**(2), 128-133.

Chapter 6

Key Management Indicators: Using Insurance Claims and Employee Survey Data

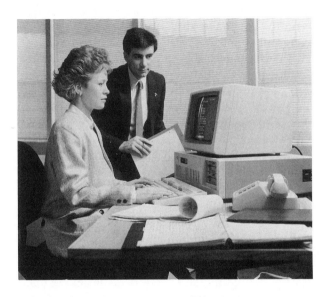

Jeffrey S. Harris
Kenneth A. Theriault

Insurance claims data linked to surveys, health risk appraisals, payroll and personnel information, and other relevant records can be used for ongoing management assessment of the effects of health promotion programs, if data are adjusted properly and if their basic accuracy and constraints are appreciated. The specific indicators should be agreed on in advance to avoid later debates and searches for information. Similarly, data collection systems should be established as an initial component of health promotion and disease prevention programs, and the content and quality of claims data should be assessed initially and improved if necessary. Health promotion programs should be held to the same standards of accountability as other business or organizational functions, particularly if there is cost pressure or a change of management. Administrators who use management indicators to continually improve the performance of their programs are in the best position to maximize the benefits produced for the organization, ensuring that that stream of benefits continues.

Selecting Key Management Indicators

Managers of organizations need information to monitor, track, and direct activities under their control. As many students of management have learned, "You can't manage what you can't measure." Good management practice also dictates that each activity should periodically be quantitatively reevaluated to make sure that it is contributing to the success of the organization. But what does "contributing to the success of the organization" mean? In general, it means that the activity demonstrably influences the attainment of one or more organizational goals. The business rationale for an organization to support health promotion should be that it furthers those goals and objectives. So health promotion program and general managers must agree on and use a specific, easily obtainable, and congruent set of measures to determine the benefit of the program.

Many practitioners of health promotion would like company support for their activities because they are "the right thing to do" for employees. However, even if an activity is desirable from a preventive, ethical, or humanitarian standpoint, if it does not contribute to either the long- or short-run success of the company or nonprofit organization, management might well question why it is being funded. Therefore, in designing management indicators and the data systems to produce those indicators, the health promotion officer must show clearly how each measurement demonstrates program support of the organizational mission and goals in a strategic management context.

The Strategic Health Promotion Planning Process

Mapping program goals and objectives onto organizational objectives is a key part of the strategic management of health. Strategic health management is a data-driven, long-range, inclusive approach based on the concept that, on both an individual and a group basis, health is not a matter of chance but is something that can be managed through health promotion, detection of disease, properly designed benefits programs, early and cost-effective treatment, and rapid rehabilitation, if necessary. It clearly goes beyond the limits of post hoc diagnosis and treatment and well beyond conventional indemnity reimbursement. Strategic health management uses the tools of planning, budgeting, directing, marketing, evaluation, and organizational design to take more control of health and the costs associated with maintaining it. This chapter focuses on the measurement of the impact of this process.

Potential Indicators

There are several candidates for bottom-line measures to track and evaluate health promotion programs at the workplace, shown in Table 6.1. More information on the specific metrics for the first three indicators is available in publications on benefits data analysis (Harris, 1992b).

Note that all of these measures are *rates*. The use of rates rather than absolute numbers is important in an era of rapid growth or downsizing of many organizations. Though some managers insist on looking at absolute numbers, relative measures, such as rates per employee or cost as a percentage of income, are important to understanding the effect that an activity is having. In fact, when making internal investments, managers

Table 6.1
Potential Sources of Health Promotion Data

Indicator	Possible source
Cost of medical benefits per employee or per participant and nonparticipant	Medical insurance claims
Volume of medical services used (both inpatient and outpatient)	Medical insurance claims
Price of medical services or groups of services used to treat a specific problem	Medical insurance claims
Disability income payments per employee	Payroll system
Workers' compensation payments per employee	Risk management information system
Turnover rates	Human resource information system (HRIS)
Absence from work	Payroll or HRIS
Productivity measures	Operations
Health risk factors	Health risk appraisals Surveys
Recruitment rates	Staffing department

frequently use percentages (e.g., hurdle rates) to decide whether an activity should be done. Such measures can be called "bottom-line outputs." That is, they have a direct impact on the profitability of corporations or the ability of nonprofit organizations to meet their budgets.

Some intermediate variables can also be evaluated. These include health status and quantified health risk levels. It is important to make the connection, in a quantified way, between risk levels, health status, and pooled cost over a certain period. Many organizational managers have made the point that they are not in the business of improving health; they are in the business of producing a product or providing a service. In this context, health status and risk level are important, but only because they lead to one of the outcome measures mentioned.

Finally, one could look at what might be called primary variables. Many health promotion programs have been, and still are, evaluated on the basis of changes in attitudes, changes in beliefs, job satisfaction, satisfaction with program activities, and morale. These measures are generally determined from surveys. Though these may intuitively support the productivity of an organization, unless a clear connection can be made between these variables and changes in health or risk and financially quantifiable measurements, they are not relevant in the final analysis to the conduct of health promotion programs in work organizations. If beliefs are evaluated, they should be beliefs that have been clearly shown to contribute to employees' or dependents' ability to improve their health habits or health status, such as locus of control and self-efficacy.

Programs have also been evaluated on the basis of participation rates. Although participation may apparently justify the existence of fixed assets such as fitness centers, participation per se is actually a use of time rather than a payback on assets or investment.

Data Capture and Information Systems

The selection of management indicators for health promotion program effectiveness is dependent on what information is being routinely captured and stored in the various data systems to which management has access. These include the medical claims processing, personnel (i.e., payroll and attendance data), health promotion program, employee assistance program, and utilization management systems. The data typically captured in medical claims systems have already been described.

Most employers have computerized systems for payroll activities. These systems typically provide information about an employee's date of birth, sex, marital status, salary, job category, date of hire, status (full-time or part-time), and medical coverage selection. Some systems also record ethnicity, level of education, and absenteeism information. Fewer systems track absenteeism by category or reason for absence (vacation, illness, discipline, leave of absence, etc.). For some employers such records are not computerized but exist only on paper in employee personnel files.

Where companies have health promotion programs in place, they may or may not have computerized systems implemented to monitor these programs and employees' participation in them. When systems do exist, they typically record various dates, including date of initial contact, health assessment or health risk appraisal, class participation, follow-up contacts, and so on. Some systems also record basic health information (e.g., height, weight, blood pressure). Others integrate more detailed health history information obtained via a comprehensive health risk appraisal; often, however, the HRA data are in a separate system.

Systems for monitoring employee assistance program (EAP) participation rates and effectiveness are mentioned here because of the cross-referral that can and should occur between an employer's EAP and health promotion programs. These typically record an employee identifier, contact and follow-up dates, nature and severity of the presenting problem, the assistance recommended or provided by the counselor, and basic outcome information (e.g., improved, resolved, or unchanged). In some systems, particularly those in which the EAP serves as a gatekeeper in a comprehensive managed mental health program, data about the provider, cost, and type of mental health services provided are also collected.

Utilization management systems, sometimes maintained by the insurer or other third party administrator but often by an independent utilization management firm, typically provide information concerning the precertification of inpatient hospitalizations and continued hospital stay, such as diagnosis, date of certification, number of days requested, number of days approved, next review date, and provider names. Some also track precertification information for outpatient surgical services or expensive medical procedures. Others record the activities of individual case management programs, but this information is frequently narrative in form and thus not easily included in a computer-based analysis.

The information available from medical and workers' compensation claims can be matched for each employee with data from surveys and the human resource and payroll systems to create a more complete picture of each episode of ill health or absence from work. We will concentrate on the utility of claims data, because the analysis of the other data is more straightforward. However, it is important to make the linkage *if* one claims that by reducing ill health, risk reduction activities were responsible for an employee's greater availability for work. If total availability (i.e., lack of absence) is used, other variables such as morale may be responsible. This would then be a psychologically rather than a physically linked effect.

Insurance Claims Data

Insurance claims data are generally available and accessible to trained analysts and quantify the financial impact of ill health on an employer.

Claims data can be used, with a substantial number of caveats, to track an organization's expenditures for medical care over time. It is important to understand exactly what is available in claims data, what some of the inaccuracies and inexactness in the data are, what the data were designed for, and other confounding factors that may obscure the effect of health promotion programs on health service use and costs.

Claims data, typically available on magnetic tape or diskette from insurers or third-party administrators (TPAs), effectively describe a population's use of medical services and the cost of services used. For each item of service provided to an individual, the claim data will usually provide information about the patient, the provider, and the service itself (see Table 6.2). Note that until recently, such data were available from indemnity insurers but not generally from managed care organizations.

The quality of available claim data varies among insurers and TPAs, both in terms of completeness and accuracy, and translating the payer's coded information into useful categories for analysis can be difficult. Further, not all of the services provided to a particular patient may be known to the claim payer or recorded in the claim data: Claims may have been filed under a spouse's health insurance plan; a claim may not have

Table 6.2
Typical Claims Tapes Data Elements

Data describing . . .	Typically includes . . .
The patient	Identification number (encoded) Age Sex Relationship to employee (self, spouse, dependent) Diagnosis (one or more, coded)
The provider	Type of provider (hospital, physician, chiropractor, pharmacy, etc.) Provider identification number Geographic location (ZIP or postal code)
The service	Date(s) of service Setting of care (inpatient hospital, surgery center, physician office, etc.) Type of service (room & board, physician visit, lab, X-ray, etc.) Number of services (days, visits, anesthesia units, etc.) Medical or surgical procedure(s) performed (coded) Cost of service (amount charged and amount paid)

been filed at all, because the deductible had not yet been satisfied; or the provider may not have generated a bill for the service. The issues surrounding the correct use and interpretation of medical claims data are sufficiently complex to warrant the involvement of benefits consultants who have expertise in the analysis of medical benefit design and utilization.

Insurance claims data and systems were designed to track payments to providers of medical care. As already stated, these data typically contain patient identifiers, provider identifiers (which are often tax numbers only or names that do not identify exactly what the providers do or what their specialty is), the amount paid, the procedure or treatment for which payment was made, and often the provider's diagnosis. It was customary in the past, and continues widely today, to do a minimal amount of coding. Thus, it is not uncommon to find a diagnosis coded as "heart disease," which is not specific enough to determine the attributable life-style proportion. It is also common to pay claims for tests and procedures without a Current Procedural Terminology (CPT) code to specifically identify the service performed. This degree of imprecision makes it difficult to make a direct link between what is known about the effects of lifestyle and what health care services were rendered. In addition, a number of claims payers use relatively uneducated or unskilled employees to pay claims. It is often difficult for someone with a high school education to determine proper diagnostic coding based on the information provided. This situation may be improving; as of January 1, 1991, the federal government requires accurate diagnostic and procedural coding for payment of Medicare bills. This should affect all coding and record keeping.

Analytic Strategies and Issues

From 5% to 30% of claims are allocated to the "ill-defined complaints" category rather than to other major diagnostic categories. This category includes complaints that physicians were unable to diagnose, such as chest pain or back pain, but could also include fairly esoteric diagnoses or those that the claims handlers simply did not understand. It is very important to understand the content of that category to determine how much data has become unusable. If the category only contains undiagnosable complaints, it may be amenable to self-care education.

It should be obvious that one should evaluate specific diagnoses that are clearly linked to the risk factors addressed by specific health promotion programs (see Table 6.3). If one has a hypertension control program, one should look at the cluster of ICD-9 diagnoses that specifically name hypertension. One might also look at consequences of hypertension, such as specific diagnoses for kidney disease, stroke, ischemic heart disease, and hypertensive heart disease. However, examining all heart disease or

Table 6.3
Probable Short-Term Benefits of Health Promotion Activities

Activity	Reduction in
Smoking cessation	URIs
	Pneumonia
	Asthma
	Bronchitis
	Sinusitis
	Low birth-weight premature births
	Otitis and URIs in dependent children
	Sudden cardiac deaths
Cessation of heavy drinking	Trauma and domestic violence
	Seizures
	Nutritionally related disease
	Dependent use of health service
Self-care counseling or classes	Medical services for minor complaints
Wise-use classes, counseling, or hotlines	Ambulatory care and emergency room use
	Elective surgery
	Diagnostic testing
	Medication costs
Immunizations	Influenza
	Pneumonia
	Tetanus
Cardiac and neurologic rehabilitation	Absence
	Total cost
	Retraining
	Replacement
Diabetes education and control	Ketoacidosis
	Hypoglycemia
Seat belt safety	Motor vehicle trauma
Workplace and home safety	Trauma

Note. From "The Cost Effectiveness of Health Promotion Programs" by J.S. Harris. In *Managing Employee Health Care Costs: Assuring Quality and Value* (p. 168) by J.S. Harris, H.D. Belk, and L.W. Wood (Eds.), 1992, Beverly, MA: OEM Health. Copyright 1992 by Jeffrey S. Harris. Reprinted by permission.

all kidney disease would be widening the scope to the extent that any effect would probably not be apparent.

Establishing a long-term trend is important. Year to year, costs can fluctuate dramatically, except for very large organizations. One should look for inflection points in trends at the specific times when meaningful health promotion programs were introduced. One must be very careful in this time series analysis to make correlations between changes in cost or utilization and *effective* introduction of a program. Simply announcing the program is not introduction. An inflection point occurs when a meaningful number of people become involved. Alternatively, as participation or behavior changes increase, a corresponding decrease in utilization or cost might occur. Indeed, the rates for employees may be different than those for dependents if employees were exposed to the health promotion program and dependents were not. This distinction can be useful in tracking the effects on "exposed" and "unexposed" groups. For example, in the program results reported in Figure 6.1, employees were exposed to a comprehensive health promotion program; their adjusted case rate of heart attack fell. Dependents, who were not exposed directly to the program, suffered more heart attacks than did employees over 5 years.

A final caveat, which we will discuss in more detail later, regards causality versus association. If a change occurs in the level of a specific heart disease diagnosis, such as heart attack (i.e., myocardial infarction) or hypertension, after the institution of a specifically targeted health promotion program, there is still the question of whether the health promotion program caused the change or was only associated with it.

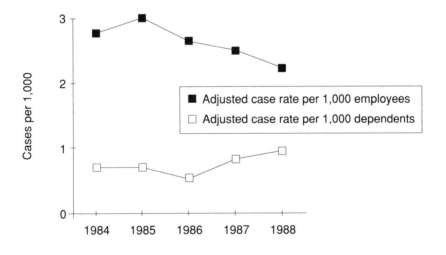

Figure 6.1   Adjusted heart attack rates per 1,000 employees and dependents. *Note.* From "A Comprehensive Approach to Health Management" by B.A. Dalton and J.S. Harris. In *Managing Employee Health Care Costs: Assuring Quality and Value* (p. 188) by J.S. Harris, H.D. Belk, and L.W. Wood (Eds.), 1992, Boston: OEM Press. Copyright 1992 by Jeffrey S. Harris. Reprinted by permission.

Adjustments to Claims Data

A number of other factors must be adjusted for before any reasonable association can be documented. These include the following:

- *Population aging.* A number of studies done by the Health Care Financing Administration and Blue Cross/Blue Shield have shown that, in the middle-aged years, for every year of increase of the average age of the population, the use of health services increases between 2.5% and 5% (Arnett, McKusick, Sonnefeld, & Cowell, 1986; Fisher, 1980; Jones, 1985). This, of course, is in a population that does not have access to a health promotion program. In theory, that curve could be flattened if increasing age had no effect on health risks. However, it is important to adjust the baseline and trend to account for aging. Otherwise, the effects of health promotion may be masked by the generally upward trend. Although the slope of the trend may have decreased, managers are apt to ask where the predicted *decrease* in costs is. Adjustment for aging makes the information easier to understand. The most effective way to age adjust, although the most complex and expensive, is to make this correction on a case-by-case basis.

- *Migration to managed care programs.* Analyses using insurance data are typically performed on claims for indemnity, or fee-for-service, insurance. However, in recent years, managed care has grown dramatically, sometimes reaching between 40% and 80% of the population of a company or nonprofit organization. Managed care organizations, in general, have not kept extensive records of claims payments. Independent practice associations (IPAs), which must pay fee-for-service or contracted fees to their practitioners, are more likely to have claims data that can be merged and analyzed with indemnity data. Typically, staff model organizations have not kept cost or volume data.

The implication of the growth of managed care for data analysis is related to who joins managed care organizations. It appears that in the earlier stages of the introduction of managed care, employees who do not have a relationship with a physician, or who are new to the area, or who are about to have children or have small children who require preventive services prefer to join staff model managed care organizations to increase their ease of access to the system and the comprehensiveness of the coverage. Typically, these employees are younger and healthier and use fewer health services. Therefore, one may see apparent increases in health care cost among those remaining in the fee-for-service program simply because low-risk, low-cost employees have selected managed care. On the other hand, IPAs tend to attract older individuals who have established relationships with physicians because of illness *if* their physician of choice is a member of the network or IPA. In this case, indemnity costs may apparently decrease. The cause of this phenomenon is sometimes called *HMO migration*.

It is important to perform an adjustment, for example, based on evaluation of an employee's use of health services before switching from an indemnity insurance program to an HMO, to understand the relative differences between the populations. One can argue with the correction factors on the basis that people will become sick after switching to managed care and there will be regression toward the mean, but an attempt should be made to adjust the data for this change in the makeup of the insured population. There can be substantial distortion of the changes in health service use and cost, which might mask any effects that health promotion programs might have.

• *Inflation*. Applying price inflation factors to medical care data is a risky undertaking. Use of the consumer price index is clearly irrelevant to the medical care system, where open-ended funding has encouraged price increases to maintain target incomes or to increase profits for health care providers (Harris, 1990). The medical care price index is also distorted, because it includes expenditures by government entities, which now account for about 40% of all health care payments. Their payments have typically been capped by law or by budget constraints. The result is that costs tend to be shifted to the private sector (Custer, 1992). For example, if there is a 3% cap on Medicare expenditures and the cost of inputs (i.e., salaries, supplies) to hospitals or doctors' offices rises 10%, the excess cost increase will be applied to the private sector, thus significantly augmenting price increases for the private sector. There is also cost-shifting from managed care plans, which have been able to contract per diem or fee schedule rates from hospitals and physicians. The question then becomes, How does one level the playing field? The various surveys of benefits cost increases conducted by consulting firms vary widely, and there are differences between self-insured organizations, which typically manage care more aggressively, and fully insured companies, which are at risk for insurance market losses, cost shifting, taxation, and a number of other factors. Perhaps the best adjustment would be to find a survey that applies to one's particular type of organization.

• *Managed care payment methods*. As discussed previously, the better managed care organizations contract for a fixed price per day with hospitals and a fee schedule, which must be renegotiated rather than simply inflated every year to control and manage the price factor of the price/volume relationship. Unfortunately, the typical consequence is that providers inflate the prices to their remaining fee-for-service patients, rather than improve the efficiency of their offices or adopt new ways of doing things. In addition, problems can be created if one tries to merge claims tapes from an IPA based on discounts, fee schedules, or per diems, with indemnity payments, which are simply payment of submitted bills subject to a profile cap.

• *Access to managed care.* If an organization has a significant number of employees in a managed care organization, which, through queuing or other means, limits access to care, it is possible that employees could become sicker and, therefore, cause increased health care costs. It is also possible that the volume of services might drop. However, this would not be due to the health promotion effort but to the restriction of access.

One should attempt to use aggregated, payment-form adjusted data from all health care providers, including managed care and indemnity plans. If this is done, one can see the effects on the entire population. One should also determine whether a managed care plan offers health promotion activities and devise ways of taking that into account, because there may be an effect on care plan costs. Also keep in mind that managed care organizations' costs are not the same thing as indemnity costs, because there are significant cost loads in the range of 12% to 20% for marketing and internal management (Harris, in press), which are obviously unrelated to the health status of employees.

• *Medical management.* One of the chief confounders of tracking health care costs and volume, besides the introduction of managed care, is utilization review. Frequently, organizations will introduce utilization review and then progressively tighten the criteria for approval of care. This causes the same effect that one might see were the level of illness to decrease in a population. It has been extremely difficult to separate this effect from that of health promotion programs. One technique examines admission rates, rather than total use of hospital days or length of stay. The reason is that, until very recently, utilization management has not been particularly effective in decreasing the decision to use services, at least not inpatient services (i.e., the admission rate). It has been effective in reducing length of stay, and, therefore, overall bed days per thousand (Gray & Field, 1989). Thus, adjusted decreases in admission rates generally should be associated with some other factor, such as health promotion (Dalton & Harris, 1992).

• *Plan design changes.* Whenever copayments or deductibles are increased, there is a small but measurable decrease in the use of health services (Harris & Custer, 1992). Look for inflection points whenever plan changes are introduced. It may be possible to use data from existing studies, such as the RAND Health Insurance Experiment (Newhouse et al., 1981), to create multipliers that will correct for such predicted decreases in use. Of course, increases in copayments and deductibles should be correlated with inflation; if copayments and deductibles are simply keeping up with inflation, they probably will have little effect on employee use of medical services.

• *Presentation to management.* In the final analysis, many business managers simply wish to track a health promotion program's contribution to the bottom line. The adjustments already described may be somewhat difficult to understand, but a clear exposition of exactly what was done to the collected data to arrive at the conclusions drawn will be needed for management presentations. To the extent possible, one should use data with as few adjustments as necessary so that the program's actual impact can be more easily understood.

• *Analytic sidelights.* One possible outcome of these adjustments would be an examination of the company's benefits structure, as well as its health promotion program. One could argue that the company is losing a significant amount of money if it is paying managed care prices that are very close to indemnity prices. However, the employees in those programs may be using a fraction of the health services used by those in the indemnity program. In that case, the recommended management action might be to have only one benefits plan, which is managed, opposed to a multiplicity of confusing plans with segmented risk. This is not a health promotion intervention, but it clears the deck for cleaner data acquisition and follow-up and reveals costs of health care that the employer can manipulate, albeit with some difficulty if there is employee resistance.

Valid Uses of Adjusted Data

Having said all of this, adjusted insurance data can be used to monitor the correlations between introductions of health promotion programs or increases in participation in health promotion programs and cost or utilization rates, if diagnoses are very specific and properly coded. One might use sentinel diagnoses for identifying short-term effects. For example, if there is a decrease in the smoking rate, one should fairly quickly see a decrease in treatment costs or volume for bronchitis and pneumonia in employees and, perhaps, for asthma in dependents. There are similar diagnoses that can be used for studying the impact of various types of lifestyle programs. Again, however, the diagnosis should be very specifically related to the intervention in the desired time frame. For example, it is not reasonable to expect a decrease in the rate of ischemic heart disease immediately after the institution of exercise or smoking cessation programs. However, one might see a decrease in deaths due to cardiac electrical conduction disturbances upon institution of smoking cessation, because that effect occurs within several weeks. On the other hand, regression of atherosclerosis cannot be expected for some time. Therefore, a long follow-up is needed, and program effects should not be overstated.

Survey and Questionnaire Data

A stronger case can be made for an effective health promotion program if one can link changes in self-reported or documented health habits and risk levels and the specific claims of each person. One could then reaggregate this data to demonstrate adjusted changes in cost and utilization for groups that participated in specific health promotion activities. This may unmask an effect, although the impact on the total population may be lost in the general trend of cost increases.

These data can be gathered using either a quantified health risk appraisal or survey data. The effects of levels of risk on mortality are fairly well known and are the basis for health risk appraisals. Health risk appraisals that use a 1-to-10 scale are not useful in this activity, however. The actual level of risk or behavior should be known.

One pitfall of this approach is that many data are based on mortality rather than morbidity—useful for life insurance analysis, but not for health insurance. As much as possible, use morbidity risk ratios to make a correlation between changes in risk levels and changes in cost or use. Links can be made between health risk appraisals or surveys and claims data. They can also be made between intermediate interventions, such as employee assistance visits, and use of specifically associated services, such as outpatient or inpatient mental health care. Again, these data must be linked specifically to identified employees in order to follow their use of health services.

When distinguishing between participants and nonparticipants, it is important to identify as "participants" only those who took part in an activity related to an area in which their health risks were high. Going to a nutrition class will not necessarily decrease someone's risk from smoking. This seems elementary, but it is a flaw seen repeatedly in the literature.

It is also important to define participation as taking part in those activities that have been shown to cause changes because they constitute a sufficient "dose" of intervention. Simply taking a health risk appraisal, for example, is probably not enough of an intervention to cause a significant change in risks or costs. When subgroups take more and more classes or make more and more changes, a dose-response curve might be constructed.

Outcomes of Claims Data Analysis

Despite the many adjustments, caveats, and difficulties with claims data and risk assessment analysis, there are some areas that provide clues to the effects of worksite health promotion. Those areas are discussed in more detail here.

Adjusted Cost Trends of Sentinel Diseases

If enough data are available, adjusted costs per case or per employee, case rates, admission rates, or hospital days per 1,000 can be diagrammed to show changes over time in entire employed populations who have been exposed to a comprehensive heath promotion program. This alternative is not as specific or quite as plausible as examining the diverging trend lines among participants and nonparticipants, but it may be the only possible design if, because of intense media exposure to health promotion or heavy penetration of the population by health promotion activities, there are too few "unexposed" individuals.

For example, a study of the population of Northern Telecom, Inc. after 5 years of a comprehensive health promotion, EAP, and primary care/wise-use/self-care education program, which included significant media and peer interaction components, revealed downward trends in adjusted costs in some sentinel diseases (Dalton & Harris, 1992). The adjusted cost per case of mental health diagnoses dropped sharply. The EAP probably contributed to this effect, but it is likely that institution of a benefits cap and intensified utilization management also contributed (see Figure 6.2).

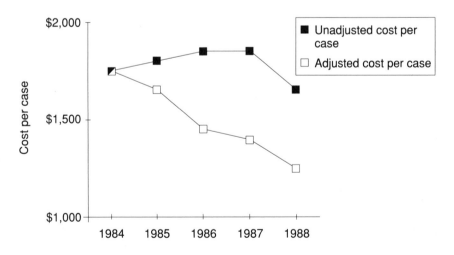

Figure 6.2   Unadjusted and adjusted costs per case for mental disorders. *Note.* From "A Comprehensive Approach to Health Management" by B.A. Dalton and J.S. Harris. In *Managing Employee Health Care Costs: Assuring Quality and Value* (p. 184) by J.S. Harris, H.D. Belk, and L.W. Wood (Eds.), 1992, Boston: OEM Press. Copyright 1992 by Jeffrey S. Harris. Reprinted by permission.

Adjusted hospitalization rates for key diagnoses also dropped (see Table 6.4). All of the listed diagnoses should have been affected by the health promotion media and the specific programs offered, which included "wise use of medical care" materials given and shown to most employees and self-care educational materials and instruction, which were widely available. This measure was sensitive to the effects of health promotion and disease prevention. A utilization management program was instituted 2 years after the health promotion program but affected mainly the length of stay rather than the number of admissions, which decreased only 1% to 2%.

The cost per case dropped compared to baseline. The data shown here are ratios, because the actual cost figures are company-confidential (see Table 6.5). The adjusted cost per 1,000 employees compared to a base year also dropped (see Table 6.6).

Comparison of employees, who were exposed to the health promotion program, and dependents, who were not, was revealing in some cases. For example, the adjusted rate of myocardial infarction (i.e., heart attack) for employees dropped over the 5-year period, whereas the rate of incidence for dependents rose (see Figure 6.1).

Table 6.4
Hospitalization Rate Decreases
for Key Diagnostic Categories and Procedures (per 1,000 Claimants)

Diagnostic category	1984	1985	1986	1987	1988
Infectious disease	1.0	1.4	1.2	1.2	0.9
Endocrine, immune disorders	1.6	1.3	1.1	1.0	1.0
Asthma, bronchitis	1.4	1.2	1.0	0.9	0.7
Gastritis, colitis	1.7	1.4	1.3	1.3	0.8
Genitourinary conditions	13.0	8.4	7.0	5.9	5.3
Female genital conditions*	18.2	12.1	10.7	8.9	8.2
Bone, connective tissue	5.7	4.7	4.1	3.1	3.1
Congenital anomaly	1.3	1.6	0.9	0.9	0.7
Injuries	4.4	5.5	5.1	4.1	3.5
Ill-defined complaints	16.7	12.0	4.7	3.8	4.0
All diagnoses	95.9	93.3	88.0	80.6	73.0

*Denominator is females over age 18 yr only.

Note. From "A Comprehensive Approach to Health Management" by B.A. Dalton and J.S. Harris. In Managing Employee Health Care Costs: Assuring Quality and Value (p. 186) by J.S. Harris, H.D. Belk, and L.W. Wood (Eds.), 1992, Beverly, MA: OEM Health. Copyright 1992 by Jeffrey S. Harris. Reprinted by permission.

Table 6.5
Cost per Case Decreases Compared to Base Year
for Key Diagnostic Categories and Procedures (per 1,000 Claimants)

Diagnostic category	1984	1985	1986	1987	1988
Infectious disease	1.00	0.84	0.85	0.84	0.80
Malignancy	1.00	0.67	0.77	0.72	0.60
Mental disorders	1.00	0.92	0.80	0.73	0.61
Substance abuse	1.00	0.92	0.80	0.73	0.61
Circulatory disease	1.00	0.94	1.07	0.45	0.50
Asthma, bronchitis	1.00	0.87	0.77	0.66	0.73
Gastritis, colitis	1.00	0.79	0.86	0.70	0.56
Genitourinary conditions	1.00	0.86	0.79	0.75	0.64
Female genital conditions*	1.00	0.93	0.85	0.80	0.73
Birth-related procedures	1.00	0.94	0.95	0.92	0.87
Skin disorders	1.00	0.94	0.79	0.75	0.73
Bone, connective tissue	1.00	0.94	0.81	0.74	0.73
Congenital anomaly	1.00	0.45	0.42	0.38	0.44
All diagnoses	1.00	0.91	0.88	0.88	0.82
All diagnoses minus births	1.00	0.88	0.83	0.84	0.78

*Denominator is females over age 18 yr only.

Note. From "A Comprehensive Approach to Health Management" by B.A. Dalton and J.S. Harris. In *Managing Employee Health Care Costs: Assuring Quality and Value* (p. 188) by J.S. Harris, H.D. Belk, and L.W. Wood (Eds.), 1992, Beverly, MA: OEM Health. Copyright 1992 by Jeffrey S. Harris. Reprinted by permission.

Adjusted Population Cost Trends Compared to Control Populations

Two plants offering the Johnson & Johnson LIVE FOR LIFE program were compared to a plant not offering the program (Bly, Jones, & Richardson, 1986). The two program sites had statistically significant lower increases in hospital admissions, bed-days, and costs over 5 years. There were no statistically significant differences for other health care costs or utilization. Interestingly, the major reason for the difference in costs was a small increase in adjusted costs in the control site in the last year of the study. It is not known if the trend continued or if it was an anomaly, because the trend line was not linear.

Adjusted Absence Rate Trends

After adjusting for age, sex, and baseline absence levels, participants of a physical fitness program at The Travelers' Taking Care Center had fewer

Table 6.6
Ratios of Cost per 1,000 Claimants to Base Year

Diagnostic category	1985	1986	1987	1988
Mental disorders	1.00	0.94	0.87	0.76
Substance abuse	1.00	0.95	0.91	0.72
Asthma, bronchitis	1.00	0.83	0.81	0.82
Ulcer	1.00	0.67	0.63	0.60
Gastritis, colitis	1.00	1.08	0.92	0.68
Female genital disorders	1.00	0.80	0.80	0.73
Birth-related procedures	1.00	1.04	0.96	0.89
Injuries				
Inpatient treatment	1.00	0.81	0.58	0.61
Outpatient treatment	1.00	1.07	0.98	0.93
Total	1.00	0.96	0.80	0.79
Ill-defined complaints	1.00	0.84	0.79	0.64
All diagnoses				
Inpatient treatment	1.00	0.98	0.90	0.78
Outpatient treatment	1.00	1.06	0.91	0.95
Total	1.00	1.02	0.91	0.87
All diagnoses minus birth-related procedures				
Inpatient treatment	1.00	0.95	0.87	0.77
Outpatient treatment	1.00	1.06	0.91	0.94
Total	1.00	1.01	0.90	0.87

Note. From "A Comprehensive Approach to Health Management" by B.A. Dalton and J.S. Harris. In *Managing Employee Health Care Costs: Assuring Quality and Value* (p. 189) by J.S. Harris, H.D. Belk, and L.W. Wood (Eds.), 1992, Beverly, MA: OEM Health. Copyright 1992 by Jeffrey S. Harris. Reprinted by permission.

absences compared to a matched population (Lynch, Golaszewski, Clearie, Snow, & Vickery, 1990). Similar results have been reported elsewhere.

Data Linkage Studies

After claims data have been adequately reviewed for accuracy and completeness, and appropriately adjusted for the statistical factors outlined previously, they can be linked to data from other sources (e.g., personnel data, program participation records, health risk appraisals, surveys, etc.) to form a composite data base. This data base can then be used to generate a variety of management indicators, which can measure program effectiveness and impact.

For example, the relationship between actual and expected health claims costs for program participants and nonparticipants can be compared over time. In one study of a major employer's health promotion program, the ratio of actual to expected health claims costs for individuals who participated in the program decreased following participation, whereas the ratio for nonparticipants increased. Table 6.7 shows these results (Alexander & Alexander, 1992).

Although participants saw a reduction in health costs and non-participants did not, it is interesting that participants and nonparticipants both had health claims costs that were below expected levels. This is likely because the population being studied were employees who had completed a health risk appraisal (HRA), a self-selected group which, on average, was healthier than the work force as a whole. This finding is itself important and useful to the management of the health promotion program.

In the same study, claims costs were analyzed for individuals whose HRA results indicated that they were heavy smokers or were at high risk for mental illness. In the 3 years before taking the HRA, these individuals had claims costs in excess of the expected levels for their age, sex, job category, years of education, and location. However, during the year in which they took the HRA and during the 2 years following, their claims costs returned to levels that were not significantly different from expected levels. Table 6.8 summarizes these results.

The figures suggest that the mere act of taking the HRA had an impact on individuals' health behaviors and, indirectly, on their medical claims costs.

Cost Distribution Studies

Several studies have measured the differences in incurred costs between low- and high-risk individuals (Brink, 1987; Yen, Eddington, & Witting,

Table 6.7
Claims Cost for Health Promotion Participants and Nonparticipants

Year	Participants' claims cost			Nonparticipants' claims cost		
	Actual	Expected	Ratio	Actual	Expected	Ratio
1	$1,642	$3,192	0.51	$1,038	$3,065	0.34
2	$1,369	$2,883	0.47	$1,313	$2,981	0.44

Note. Data from *McDonnell Douglas Health Promotion Effectiveness Study,* by Alexander and Alexander Consulting Group, 1992, unpublished study.

Table 6.8
Excess Claims Costs by Risk Factor

Risk category	Excess costs		
	During 3 yr before HRA	During 1 yr after HRA	During 2 yr after HRA
Smoking	$585	$0	$0
Mental illness	$312	$0	$0

Note. Data from McDonnell Douglas Health Promotion Effectiveness Study, by Alexander and Alexander Consulting Group, 1992, unpublished study.

1991). They revealed either bimodal distributions of risk and cost or continuously related curves. In a bimodal distribution, those with low risks accrue low costs, and those with high risks accrue high costs. The continuously related curve was a dose-response curve, with progressively higher costs as risks increase. Though these studies add a cost dimension to epidemiologic work, which demonstrated dose-response curves between risk and disease, they do not show an effect of health promotion over time. They are baseline, or cross-sectional, information.

Evaluation Studies

Periodic evaluations of health promotion programs, which may be more rigorous than ongoing management accounting, should meet more comprehensive design and adjustment criteria than those described in this discussion. A list of these criteria appears in Table 6.9 (Harris, 1992b). These criteria were derived from a meta-analysis of expert suggestions offered in the literature.

Summary

Insurance claims data can be used for ongoing management assessment of the effects of health promotion programs, if adjusted properly and if the basic accuracy and constraints of the data are appreciated. Linking claims data to surveys, health risk appraisals, payroll and personnel data, and other relevant records strengthens the specific measurement or comparison. The specific indicators should be agreed on in advance, to avoid later debates and searches for information. Similarly, data collection systems should be established as a basic component of health promotion

Table 6.9
Health Promotion Evaluation Design Criteria

Clear definition of program goals, preferably agreed to by top management
Specific measurable definitions for risk factors and other outcome measures
Baseline measures of health risk, service use, and financial variables
Ability to match program exposure data, health risk data, and utilization and
    financial data for each individual
Comparison to control groups or statistical adjustment to control for baseline
    differences; cost inflation; changes in community health behaviors, medical
    practice patterns, benefits packages (e.g., introduction of utilization review)
Specific operational definitions of outcomes
Adequate sample size
Adequate time of follow-up
Appropriate analytical techniques

Note. From "The Cost Effectiveness of Health Promotion Programs" by J.S. Harris. In *Managing Employee Health Care Costs: Assuring Quality and Value* (p. 169) by J.S. Harris, H.D. Belk, and L.W. Wood (Eds.), 1992, Beverly, MA: OEM Health. Copyright 1992 by Jeffrey S. Harris. Reprinted by permission.

and disease prevention programs, and the content and quality of claims data (i.e., coding, accessibility, and completeness) should be assessed and improved, if necessary, *before* such programs begin. Health promotion programs will probably be held to the same standards of accountability as other business or organizational functions, particularly if there is cost pressure or a change of management. Program administrators who are prepared will be in the best position to maximize the benefits produced by their programs.

References

Alexander & Alexander Consulting Group. (1992). *McDonnell Douglas health promotion effectiveness study.* Unpublished study.

Arnett, R.H., McKusick, D.R., Sonnefeld, S.T., & Cowell, C.S. (1986). Projections of health care spending to 1990. *Health Care Financing Review, 7,* 1-36.

Bly, J.L., Jones, R.C., & Richardson, J.E. (1986). Impact of worksite health promotion on health care costs and utilization: Evaluation of Johnson & Johnson's LIVE FOR LIFE program. *Journal of the American Medical Association, 256,* 3235-3240.

Brink, S.D. (1987). *Health risks and behavior: The impact of medical costs.* Milwaukee: Milliman & Robertson.

Custer, W.S. (1992). Health care cost inflation and employer cost management. *Journal of Occupational Medicine, 32*(12), 1229-1234.

Dalton, B.A., & Harris, J.S. (1992). A comprehensive approach to corporate health management. In J.S. Harris, H.D. Belk, & L.W. Wood (Eds.), *Managing employee health care costs: Assuring quality and value* (pp. 181-191). Boston: OEM Health.

Fisher, C.R. (1980). Differences by age groups in health care spending. *Health Care Financing Review, 1*, 65-90.

Gray, B.H., & Field, M.J. (1989). *Controlling costs and changing patient care? The role of utilization management.* Washington, DC: National Academy Press.

Harris, J.S. (1992a). Why doctors do what they do: Determinants of physician behavior. In J.S. Harris, H.D. Belk, & L.W. Wood (Eds.), *Managing employee health care costs: Assuring quality and value* (pp. 57-70). Boston: OEM Health.

Harris, J.S. (1992b). Watching the numbers: Basic data for health care management. In J.S. Harris, H.D. Belk, & L.W. Wood (Eds.), *Managing employee health care costs: Assuring quality and value* (pp. 100-103). Boston: OEM Health.

Harris, J.S. (in press). *Strategic health management.* San Francisco: Jossey-Bass.

Harris, J.S., & Custer, W.S. (1992). Health care economic factors and the effects of benefits plan design changes. In J.S. Harris, H.D. Belk, & L.W. Wood (Eds.), *Managing employee health care costs: Assuring quality and value* (pp. 108-115). Boston: OEM Health.

Jones, S.P. (1985). The costs of membership aging in a Blue Cross and Blue Shield plan. *Inquiry, 22*, 201-205.

Lynch, W.D., Golaszewski, T.J., Clearie, A.F., Snow, D., & Vickery, D.M. (1990). Impact of a facility-based corporate fitness program on the number of absences from work due to illness. *Journal of Occupational Medicine, 32*, 9-12.

Newhouse, J.P., Manning, W.G., Morris, C.N., Orr, L.L., Duan, N., Keeler, E.B., Leibowitz, A., Marquis, K.H., Marquis, M.S., Phelps, C.E., & Brook, R.H. (1981). Some interim results from a controlled trial of cost sharing in health insurance. *New England Journal of Medicine, 305*, 1501-1507.

Yen, L.T., Eddington, D.W., & Witting, P. (1991). Associations between health risk appraisal scores and employee medical claims costs in a manufacturing company. *American Journal of Health Promotion, 6*(1), 46-54.

PART III

Worksite
Health Promotion Profiles

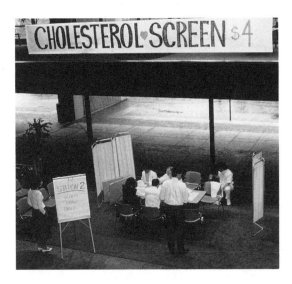

The measurement of the economic impact of worksite health promotion has been carried out in numerous settings. Although many of the most comprehensive evaluations have been done in large private corporations, the expansion of the field into virtually all work sectors has encouraged concomitant efforts to evaluate programs in these different settings. This part provides evaluations of five distinctly different types of worksite health promotion programs.

The focus in chapter 7, by Kristan Goldfein, William Schneider, and John Allegrante, is on a mammography screening program at a large financial institution. Their assessment shows the effectiveness of a highly targeted health promotion program at reducing breast cancer risk and associated health care costs.

In chapter 8, William Jose provides a comprehensive description of an increasingly popular method of holding down health care costs—risk-rated health insurance. In addition to an overview of the rationale and principles of risk-rated designs, Jose highlights a specific worksite example of the effectiveness of this cost-containment strategy.

In chapter 9, William Whitmer, James Hilyer, and Kathleen Brown review the economic impact of a worksite health promotion program for employees of the city government of Birmingham, Alabama. This unique study provides an example of the effectiveness of health promotion programs targeted at employees of local units of government.

Another significant public employee sector of the work force is America's public school systems. Todd Rogers in chapter 10 provides a cost-benefit analysis of a health promotion program at a local school district that uses a quasi-experimental method.

In chapter 11, Jonathan Fielding reviews the findings of one of the most comprehensive and well-known corporate worksite health promotion programs, the LIVE FOR LIFE program at Johnson & Johnson Corporation. LIVE FOR LIFE is a broad-based, multifactor, multisite health promotion program and provides one of the most important models in the field of worksite health promotion.

Chapter 7

Worksite Mammography Screening: The Morgan Guaranty Trust Company

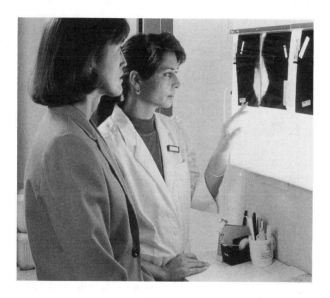

Kristan D. Goldfein
William J. Schneider
John P. Allegrante

According to Freudenheim (1992) and Geisel (1992), health expenditures represented 4.4% of the United States' gross national product (GNP) in 1950. By 1985, they represented 10.7%. Even during 1991, when the consumer price index increased by only 3.1%, medical care costs rose at a rate of 7.9%. Federal analysts estimate that by the end of 1993, national spending for medical care will have increased to approximately $940 billion (US Dept. of Commerce, 1993).

A recent survey of 2,409 companies, including both small businesses and Fortune 500 corporations, reveals how burdened American businesses have become by such increases. The survey conducted by New York's A. Foster Higgins and Co. (1992) found that group health care costs rose 18.6% in 1988, 16.7% in 1989, and 17.1% in 1990. Between 1990 and 1991 total health care costs per employee increased 12.1%, the lowest increase reported since 1986. And still, this increase was four times greater than the cost of living that year. Thus, in just 6 years, total health care costs per employee increased by 109.1%, from $1,724 in 1985 to $3,605 in 1991.

Although there is an absence of well-designed empirical studies that have demonstrated the economic merits of worksite health promotion (Warner, 1987; Warner, Wickizer, Wolfe, Schildroth, & Samuelson, 1988), prevention nonetheless is viewed by many employers as a better means than treatment of reducing medical expenses. Consequently, during the last decade many employers have turned their attention to implementing and institutionalizing worksite health promotion programs to educate and assist their employees to adopt healthful lifestyles.

Employers have supported such programs since the 1920s (Powell, 1992). Health screening, employee assistance, and health education programs also were common throughout the 1950s (Fuchs & Richards, 1985). However, the surge of employer interest in wellness and fitness programs is a relatively recent development. Pushed along by national policy interest in health promotion and disease prevention, worksite health promotion programs became more popular during the late 1970s and throughout the 1980s. In 1989, 17% of all businesses offered health promotion programs. In 1990 that figure increased to 27%, then to 32% in 1991 (Powell, 1992). According to the National Survey of Worksite Health Promotion Activities, 66% of worksites with more than 50 employees have at least one health promotion activity, with the most frequently identified programs being smoking control, health risk or health status assessment, back care, stress management, exercise and fitness, and off-the-job accident prevention (Christenson & Kiefhaber, 1988).

Health screening can be an important component of a company's approach to employee health. Screening is designed to identify risk factors for disease or to detect existing health problems during the earliest stages when individuals are asymptomatic and the underlying disease is most likely to be successfully treated (Russell, 1986). There is considerable data to show that screening for hypertension and other diseases—where early detection is both possible and reasonably inexpensive and where effective therapy exists—may be the most cost-effective health promotion activity at the worksite (Russell, 1986).

In 1986, Morgan Guaranty Trust Co. in New York City—like many business organizations—developed a series of efforts designed to improve the health of employees, while at the same time attempting to reduce its health care costs. A major focus of their efforts is screening. In this chapter we describe the comprehensive breast cancer screening and education program offered at Morgan Guaranty. We focus on the screening program to emphasize that some worksite health promotion programs do have the potential to reduce health care costs and, most importantly, contribute to saving lives.

Morgan Guaranty's Health Promotion Program

J.P. Morgan & Co., Inc., founded in 1860 by John Pierpont Morgan, is a financial firm serving corporations, governments, institutions, and individuals. Morgan employs nearly 14,000 people worldwide, with half of its employees based in New York City. The health promotion program at Morgan Guaranty was not originally developed to reduce health care costs. Rather, a change in the federal tax policy in 1984 regarding corporate medical reimbursement accounts (Internal Revenue Code, section 125) provided an opportunity to fund a comprehensive in-house health promotion program. Medical reimbursement accounts allow employees to set aside predetermined amounts of their salaries, tax-free, for anticipated medical expenses. Before 1984, unused funds in such accounts were deemed taxable and were returned to employees at the end of the year. However, in 1984 the federal government determined that all unused funds would be forfeited to the employing company. These forfeited funds from employees' medical reimbursement accounts now are used by Morgan Guaranty for its employee health promotion program, an indirect but nevertheless meaningful way of returning to employees the funds they had originally invested in their health care.

Program Organizational Format

The health promotion program at Morgan Guaranty was designed to address specific health issues at designated intervals throughout the fiscal year. The program is characterized by a repeating, 4-year cyclical format, with a broad program focus for each year (Schneider, Stewart, & Haughey, 1989). The program began in September 1986 and now is in its second cycle. The first year of the cycle, called the "Year of the Heart," focuses on the prevention of cardiovascular disease. The second year, the "Year of the Body," emphasizes the prevention and early detection of cancer. The third year, the "Year of the Mind," explores psychological and social topics, such as work-related stress, child care, depression, and substance abuse. Finally, the fourth year, the "Year of Good Health," addresses those health promotion issues that do not fall within the framework of the first 3 years (e.g., healthy pregnancy, personal safety, and diabetes management; see Figure 7.1).

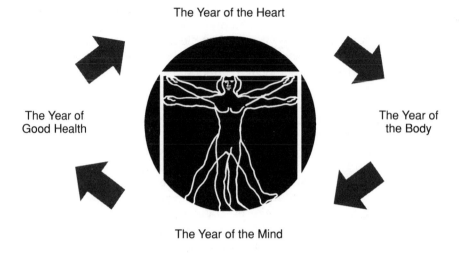

The Year of the Heart

The Year of
Good Health

The Year of
the Body

The Year of the Mind

Figure 7.1   Morgan Guaranty's 4-year cyclical program.

Each year is further subdivided into 1- or 2-month blocks. For example, during the Year of the Body, each month is dedicated to the prevention and early detection of a particular type of cancer: prostate and testicular cancer, breast cancer, lung cancer, oral cancer, colon cancer, female genital cancer, and skin cancer. AIDS also is addressed during this year, because of its similarities to neoplastic illnesses.

Program Goals and Principles

In creating the 4-year cycle, the company's medical department sought to establish certain goals and principles for the program. The program was designed to be thoroughly comprehensive without obscuring more relevant issues by directing concomitant attention to others. Similarly, the program was designed to address topics sequentially so that it would not drain the medical department of its resources. Regular revisits to each broad component serve both to reinforce the importance of particular health habits and practices and to incorporate the most recent medical developments. However, there is also a program option that allows topics of demonstrated interest and need to be included, even if such efforts extend beyond the originally designated time allotment.

The Mammography Screening Program at Morgan Guaranty

Though many of the individual components of the program have been successful in meeting their goals, the mammography breast cancer screening program, initiated in 1991 during the second Year of the Body, specifically demonstrates the potential of worksite screening programs both to reduce medical costs and to contribute to prolonging the lives of employees. This program also reveals the importance of identifying issues of need, not just those of interest, when planning any program.

As more women enter the workforce, employers cannot afford to underestimate the importance of breast cancer screening programs. Breast cancer is the most common malignancy in American women today. It is the number 2 killer, after lung cancer, of all women over age 35, and the incidence of breast cancer is rising in all age categories (American Cancer Society, 1992). In 1970, 1 in 13 women was affected by the disease. Today, 1 in 9 women is affected. The American Cancer Society (1992) estimated that in 1992, 181,000 new cases of breast cancer would be detected and 46,300 individuals (46,000 women and 300 men) would die from the disease.

Mammography is the best available screening method by which breast cancer can be detected in its early stages (Forrest & Aitken, 1990). It is the only screening modality with the potential for detecting breast cancer in a nonpalpable, highly curable stage. Unfortunately, many studies indicate that mammography is underutilized (Hamwi, 1990; McLelland, 1991; Metropolitan Life Insurance Company, 1991). According to Haynes, Odenkirchen, and Heimendinger (1990) and McLelland (1990), if mammography screening were more widely used, it could significantly reduce the overall mortality from breast cancer. Clearly, employers are in a unique position to inform their employees of the benefits of mammography and to improve the accessibility and quality of comprehensive breast cancer education and screening services.

Program Description

The 1991 screening mammography program at Morgan Guaranty incorporated several operational components.

Lectures, Workshops, and Screenings.   Education is an important component of any worksite health promotion program. Education can alleviate fear of the unknown and help employees develop a sense of control, while providing up-to-date information on medical advancements and physician recommendations (Fernsler, 1989). In 1991 during our second Year of the Body, free educational sessions focusing on breast self-examination and the importance of breast cancer screening were offered during the lunch hour to all employees. Printed educational materials and training sessions also were offered to encourage practice of breast self-examination and mammography at regular, recommended intervals. Screening mammography was offered on-site, both in vans and in nearby offices, either without charge or for a nominal fee. Guidelines suggested by the American Cancer Society and the National Cancer Institute were followed to determine those women who were eligible to participate in the mammography program.

Program Publicity.   Publicity for the program was extensive. A health newsletter written by medical department personnel was sent by internal mail to every employee. Individual letters accompanied by relevant brochures also were sent to all women employees 35 years of age and older, and posters were strategically placed throughout company facilities.

Computerized Tracking System.   Obtaining follow-up information after abnormal interpretations is an important aspect of any mammography program, but it can be tedious and time-consuming and produce suboptimal results (Monticciolo & Sickles, 1990; Sickles, 1990). Consequently, Morgan Guaranty developed a computerized tracking system to facilitate the operation and management of the program. This system performs several invaluable services, including maintenance of a data base of examination records, facilitation of tracking follow-up procedures, and provision of comprehensive program reports. Of particular concern in establishing the program was that women who had received inconclusive mammography reports might not seek the recommended follow-up procedures; using the computer system, these women could be easily identified and encouraged to complete their examinations.

Program Results

In 1991, 525 women participated in the program and six early cancers were identified and excised. On the basis of the percentage of eligible employees who participated, this was Morgan Guaranty's most successful health promotion program. Many women who underwent mammography had never before undergone the procedure.

Of the 525 reports generated by the screening program, 368 negative reports were returned. Various kinds of follow-up were proposed for the remaining 157 inconclusive reports, including repeat mammography (59), comparison views with earlier X-rays (27), compression or magnification views (26), clinical exam (21), biopsy (12), and sonogram (12). Twenty-nine of the 157 women who had received inconclusive reports were advised to have multiple follow-up studies (see Figure 7.2).

Program Costs

Several direct and indirect costs to the company and to the participants are inherent to a screening mammography program.

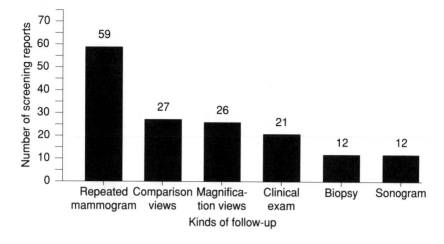

Figure 7.2   Disposition of inconclusive mammography screening results ($n =$ 157). Of the 525 women screened, 368 had mammogram results that were negative.

Operational and Administrative Costs

Costs incurred by the company for running the program were minimal and included expenses for staff time, office supplies, and adding the computerized tracking system to the existing computer system. On-site mammography was offered free of charge to all employees by a health maintenance organization (HMO) to which a number of the employees subscribe. Though the availability of free mammography is unusual, low-cost mammography is generally accessible and, indeed, has been utilized by Morgan Guaranty in other initiatives. Various operational responsibilities were distributed among regular medical staff members such that no individual would be distracted from his or her other responsibilities. Table 7.1 shows how such responsibilities were delegated among the medical department's personnel, the in-house communications department, and the health maintenance organization. All of the resources listed were critical to the success of the program.

Other Company Costs

As a result of the screening program, 2 of the 6 women diagnosed with cancer underwent mastectomy and experienced periods of disability extending to several months; the remainder were treated by lumpectomy. All 6 returned to unrestricted employment. The direct costs of breast cancer to the company included salaries to the absent employees, medical

Table 7.1
Responsibilities of Mammography Program Staff

Personnel	Program responsibilities
Medical director	Review reports Review mammography films Generate follow-up letters
Physician staff	Provide clinical breast exams
Nursing staff	Provide lectures on breast cancer Provide workshops on breast self-exams Provide counseling and support Educate employees individually & in groups Encourage program participation
Secretarial staff	Schedule mammography appointments Prepare mammography reports Prepare reminder letters
Lab technician	Review mammography reports Review mammography films
Radiologist	Interpret inconclusive films
Health education specialist	Distribute free literature Plan and publicize program Enter results into computerized data base Follow-up on pending exams
Communications department	Develop internal newsletter Develop publications Develop posters
Health maintenance organization	Provide on-site mammograms

expenses, and rehabilitation costs. Indirect costs included the inconvenience to others and disorganization during absence from work, cost of temporary replacement or overtime pay to cover the responsibilities of the absent employee, training of temporary replacements, and associated administrative costs. If any of the women had developed permanent disability or died, additional indirect costs would have included recruiting, selecting, and hiring a permanent replacement. It should be noted that screening only advances the time of disease detection and that these costs would likely be far greater in cases of more advanced illness.

Follow-Up Studies

During the program, 43% of all participants were advised to have follow-up examinations, such as short-interval mammograms, sonograms, magnification or compression mammography, and biopsy. Eight percent required multiple kinds of follow-up. In addition to medical expenses, costs included time lost due to screening and costs of evaluating false positive mammograms. Much of this cost was borne by company-sponsored, contributing health insurance.

Clinical Breast Examinations

Every woman in need of a mammogram also is in need of clinical examination of her breasts by a qualified professional. During this screening program, Morgan Guaranty's medical department offered free clinical breast examinations to all women employees; however, many women chose, for personal reasons, to be examined by outside professionals, thus incurring additional costs.

Emotional Costs

The emotional impact of receiving a mammography report, however benign the findings, can be substantial. Even reports of benign lesions—or a physician's commentary about normal breast architecture—when included in a mammogram report can be disconcerting, particularly if there is a delay in making the report available to the woman. Inconclusive reports that suggest a need for follow-up studies can be so vexing that they cause some women most in need of follow-up intervention to delay because of denial or fear. Thus, it is incumbent upon program directors to be sensitive to the emotional impact of mammography reports and ensure that reports are written clearly and with care.

Predicted Company Savings

Benefits of the program may include a reduction in mortality, morbidity, and years of productive life lost or an enhancement of quality of life, financial savings, and days of work saved (Eley, 1989). However, the number of lives saved is an obvious benefit of a screening program that detects a potentially fatal disease *only* if the screening program detects individuals in a more treatable phase or in an identifiable preclinical state (Eley, 1989). Mammography is the only modality with the potential for detecting a breast cancer while it is nonpalpable and at a stage of high curability (Hamwi, 1990). When detected early, the disease responds exceptionally well to treatment. If treated before the cancerous cells have spread, chances of complete recovery are at least 91%. Early detection of breast cancer has reduced the death rate by almost one third. Without screening programs, undetected breast cancers may become life-threatening (Forrest & Aitken, 1990).

In addition, there is growing evidence to show that health promotion programs can have a positive impact on more indirect productivity measures, such as reduced absenteeism (less time away from the job because of the convenience of the on-site facility and fewer sick days; Bertera, 1990; Lynch, Golaszewski, Clearie, Snow, & Vickery, 1990), reduced turnover, increased productivity (Leutzinger & Blanke, 1991), and increased morale (Allegrante & Michela, 1990; Gebhardt & Crump, 1990). Corporate health promotion programs also offer an opportunity for employees to feel that the company cares for their health and well-being (Owen & Long, 1989).

Consistent with the findings from recent studies (e.g., Bly, Jones, & Richardson, 1986; Gibbs, Mulvaney, Henes, & Reed, 1985; Lynch, Teitelbaum, & Main, 1992), the potential financial benefits of this screening program also included reduction in health care costs and disability payments achieved through less radical treatment of earlier stage tumors and decreased costs related to hiring and training new employees. Furthermore, the company directly benefits from the continued productivity of women who are able to stay in the work force (Eley, 1989).

The authors acknowledge, however, that screening programs may be costly in the long run, depending on the employee population. For example, a screening may detect a problem, and the company may pay for the employee's treatment. If the employee then leaves the company after receiving the medical care, the costs incurred may outweigh the economic benefits. Thus a high turnover rate may reduce the amount of cost savings.

Lessons Learned

Often, the only way to understand and appreciate the nuances of a program is to conduct one. The breast cancer screening program at Morgan Guaranty Trust provided several important insights.

First, on-site screening programs work to reduce potential barriers to proper preventive health behavior by reducing cost, inconvenience, and time lost to the employee, thereby encouraging participation. Second, although the company initially questioned the use of a mobile van unit to deliver mammography at Morgan Guaranty, because of concern that women would be deterred from using such a publicly visible facility, this was not the case. Although some women may have been discouraged by this approach, the high numbers of those who did utilize this service demonstrated its value. Moreover, the visibility of the mobile van unit had the effect of encouraging other women to inquire about participation. Of course, because mammography equipment can vary in quality, it is important to ensure that all providers use state-of-the-art equipment and have capable personnel.

Third, our experience, as well as that of others, suggests that program participants should pay at least a nominal registration fee for mammography or any other screening program. When a program is offered without charge, registrants tend to be less motivated to keep their scheduled appointment than if a fee, however small, is charged. We found that without the impetus of a token fee, many employees missed their scheduled appointments, resulting in inefficient utilization of staff and equipment. Anecdotal evidence, moreover, suggests that employees tend to value and appreciate a program more if they are required to contribute financially to it.

Fourth, a simple, inexpensive microcomputer program and tracking system can significantly assist in the operation and management of a screening program such as this. This kind of system enables more timely intervention by easily identifying women who do not comply with follow-up recommendations; thus, medical personnel were able to encourage these women to follow up. Computerized analysis of data generated by the program also can be completed more rapidly, more reliably, and at lower cost than analysis by any other method.

Finally, mammography should be offered as a continuing initiative in any worksite health promotion program. Although the recommended interval for mammography is generally 1 to 2 years for women over age 40, over two thirds of these women do not seek out these procedures. Company-sponsored programs improve the accessibility and utilization rates of comprehensive breast cancer screening services by working women, while educating and encouraging these women to use them.

Summary

Comprehensive worksite health promotion programs need to improve the availability, accessibility, and quality of breast cancer screening and educational services to address the growing needs of the increasing number of women in the work force. Not only do such screening programs effectively communicate employers' concern about the welfare of their employees, but they also provide employers with an excellent opportunity to play a role in reducing the morbidity and mortality associated with breast cancer in women.

Despite the costs inherent in any company-sponsored screening program, employers can reduce their long-term direct and indirect medical costs by offering screening programs to their employees. Moreover, the overall benefits of risk factor identification and early cancer detection are likely to be viewed as more than compensating for the costs and obligations of such a program. In our experience, six early tumors were identified at Morgan Guaranty Trust Company in 1991. Had these not been detected, the personal impact could have been devastating, and the additional cost of treatment incurred by the medical benefits program would have been substantial. Were all of the women screened in the program to have had similar interventions elsewhere, the total direct expenditures would have been greater and the indirect costs of visiting more distant diagnostic facilities would have been incurred. Finally, by making mammography easily accessible and routine, the program educated women who are employed at Morgan Guaranty about both the value and safety of the procedure itself.

References

A. Foster Higgins & Co., Inc. (1992). *Health benefits survey 1991*. New York: Author.

American Cancer Society. (1992). *Cancer facts and figures*. Atlanta: Author.

Allegrante, J.P., & Michela, J.L. (1990). Impact of a school-based workplace health promotion program on morale of inner-city teachers. *Journal of School Health*, **60**, 25-28.

Bertera, R.L. (1990). The effects of workplace health promotion on absenteeism and employment costs in a large industrial population. *American Journal of Public Health*, **80**, 1101-1105.

Bly, J.L., Jones, R.C., & Richardson, J.E. (1986). Impact of worksite health promotion on health care costs and utilization. *Journal of the American Medical Association*, **256**, 3235-3240.

Christenson, G.M., & Kiefhaber, A. (1988). Highlights from the national survey of worksite health promotion activities. *Health Values*, **12**, 29-33.

Eley, J.W. (1989). Analyzing costs and benefits of mammography screening in the workplace. *American Association of Occupational Health Nurses Journal*, **37**, 171-177.

Fernsler, J.I. (1989). Employee counseling with respect to lifestyles, life events, and breast cancer risks. *American Association of Occupational Health Nurses Journal*, **37**, 158-165.

Forrest, A.P., & Aitken, R.J. (1990). Mammography screening for breast cancer. *Annual Review of Medicine*, **41**, 117-132.

Freudenheim, M. (1992, January 28). Health costs up 12.1 percent last year, a study says. *New York Times*, p. D2.

Fuchs, J.A., & Richards, J.E. (1985). The evolving concept of worksetting health promotion. *Health Values*, **9**, 3-6.

Gebhardt, D.L., & Crump, C.E. (1990). Employee fitness and wellness programs in the workplace. *American Psychologist*, **45**, 262-272.

Geisel, J. (1992, January 27). Some relief on health costs. *Business Insurance*, pp. 1, 78.

Gibbs, J.O., Mulvaney, D., Henes, C., & Reed, R. (1985). Worksite health promotion: Five-year trend in employee health care costs. *Journal of Occupational Medicine*, **27**, 826-830.

Hamwi, D.A. (1990). Screening mammography: Increasing the effort toward breast cancer detection. *Nurse Practitioner*, **15**, 27, 30-32.

Haynes, S.G., Odenkirchen, J., & Heimendinger, J. (1990). Worksite health promotion for cancer control. *Seminars in Oncology*, **17**, 463-484.

Leutzinger, J., & Blanke, D. (1991). The effect of a corporate fitness program on perceived worker productivity. *Health Values*, **15**, 20-29.

Lynch, W.D., Golaszewski, T.J., Clearie, A.F., Snow, D., & Vickery, D.M. (1990). Impact of a facility-based corporate fitness program on the number of absences from work due to illness. *Journal of Occupational Medicine*, **32**, 9-12.

Lynch, W.D., Teitelbaum, H.S., & Main, D.S. (1992). Comparing medical costs by analyzing high-cost cases. *American Journal of Health Promotion*, **6**, 206-213.

McLelland, R. (1990). Low-cost mass screening as a means of reducing overall mortality from breast cancer. *Recent Results in Cancer Research*, **119**, 53-59.

McLelland, R. (1991). Screening mammography. *Cancer*, **67**, 1129-1131.

Metropolitan Life Insurance Company. (1991). Breast cancer screening. *Statistical Bulletin*, **72**, 12-16.

Monticciolo, D.L., & Sickles, E.A. (1990). Computerized follow-up abnormalities detected at mammography screening. *American Journal of Roentgenology*, **155**, 751-753.

Owen, P., & Long, P. (1989). Facilitating adherence to ACS and NCI guidelines for breast cancer screening. *American Association of Occupational Health Nurses Journal*, **37**, 153-157.

Powell, D.R. (1992). Five characteristics of successful wellness programs. *Employee Assistance*, **4**, 36-38.

Russell, R.B. (1986). *Is prevention better than cure?* Washington, DC: Brookings Institution.

Schneider, W.J., Stewart, S.C., & Haughey, M.A. (1989). Health promotion in a scheduled, cyclical format. *Journal of Occupational Medicine*, **31**, 443-446.

Sickles, E.A. (1990). The usefulness of computers in managing the operation of a mammography screening practice. *American Journal of Roentgenology*, **155**, 755-761.

U.S. Department of Commerce. (1993). *United States' industrial outlook.* Washington, DC: Government Printing Office.

Warner, K.E. (1987). Selling health promotion to corporate America: Uses and abuses of the economic argument. *Health Education Quarterly*, **14**, 39-55.

Warner, K.E., Wickizer, T.M., Wolfe, R.A., Schildroth, J.E., & Samuelson, M.H. (1988). Economic implications of workplace health promotion programs: Review of the literature. *Journal of Occupational Medicine*, **30**, 106-112.

Chapter 8

Risk-Rated Benefits:
The Foldcraft Corporation

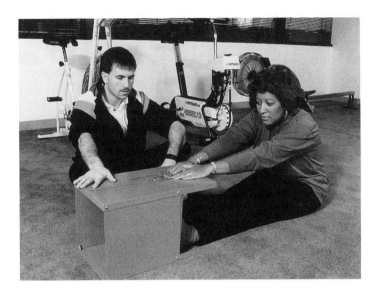

William S. Jose

Risk-rated health insurance is an increasingly attractive addition to the mix of health care benefits and cost-containment strategies in the business setting. This is in part because it is seen as an equitable way to distribute a portion of the health care cost burden and in part because it is seen as an effective way to increase consumer accountability for health care costs. A countervailing opinion, however, sees risk rating as paternal, unjustly invasive in employees' private lives, and unacceptable from a policy perspective.

I will examine here the issues involved in risk rating and make the case for investing in it as an important additional approach to coping with the health care cost crisis. Specifically, I will address the rationale for risk rating of health insurance, basic design principles for risk-rated programs, and examples of how these principles have been put into practice in a specific company.

I argue that there is a firm foundation for the implementation of risk rating from the perspective of insurance philosophy, equity in spreading the cost of health insurance, and increased accountability of all components of the health care system. I address several components and principles of plan design: organizational rewards for healthy behavior, organizational leadership, fiscal responsibility, financial incentives for employees to improve health habits, preservation of equity within the program, ethical responsibilities in program design and implementation, and reward versus punishment.

Finally, I profile the Foldcraft Corporation. Foldcraft has implemented a comprehensive risk-rating program independent of insurer involvement. Readers can judge the extent to which the program described has met the objectives and adhered to the principles I outline.

The Rationale for Risk Rating

The rationale for risk rating of health insurance is based on two principles: equity and accountability. The equity principle highlights issues related to the appropriateness of spreading the risk due to voluntarily chosen risk factors, while the accountability principle highlights issues related to the responsibility of health care consumers for a portion of the increase in health care costs.

Equity

Is it equitable for people whose voluntary lifestyle choices put them at low risk for morbidity and premature mortality to subsidize the costs of those whose voluntary lifestyle choices put them at high risk for increased morbidity and premature mortality? The idea behind the insurance concept is that the risk due to unknown or unforeseen causes should be shared among the insured group. This should not include increased risk due to voluntarily chosen risks. The consequences of any risk that is chosen by an individual ought to be borne by that individual, not subsidized by others. In the case of lifestyle risk factors, we have clear evidence that voluntary choices can create a significantly increased risk and significantly increased health care costs. Under the current system, where lifestyle risks are not factored into premium calculations, these additional, or excess, costs are borne by those whose choices have nothing to do with the increased cost and, in fact, by those whose choices actually reduce their own contribution to the collective health care cost pool. This appears to many to be an inequity.

This type of inequity does not occur in other types of insurance. In automobile insurance, for example, voluntary lifestyle behaviors that increase the risk of claims also increase the price of insurance. Breaking traffic laws—speeding, reckless driving, driving while intoxicated—are examples of individual choices that will result in higher premium costs to the insured driver. Nevertheless, the principle of paying for one's own risk has not been implemented in the area of health insurance.

Accountability

The result is a lack of accountability by the consumers of health care services. In a health care system that lacks equity, there is no incentive for the consumer to be accountable for lifestyle behaviors that can have a massive impact on health care costs. This is particularly odd in a system that calls all other actors to be accountable for their parts. Providers are urged to be accountable for appropriate, quality care. Insurers are urged to be accountable for quality and standards of care. Even researchers are urged to be more demanding when evaluating procedures of care and to expand the criteria by which alternative treatments are evaluated.

The only member of the health care system who has not been asked to cooperate in the quest to control escalating costs is the consumer. Yet, it is the consumer who is arguably the most important actor in the process. It is the consumer who ultimately makes the demand that is served by the other members of the system. This demand is clearly mediated by providers and payers, but it is first and foremost a consumer-driven demand. And in health care, the largest single determinant of consumer demand is lifestyle. High-risk lifestyle choices increase the demand for services because at-risk individuals suffer more morbidity and premature mortality than those who are not at risk. This realization should lead us to examine more closely the contribution of the consumer to the escalating crisis in health care costs and what incentives we could offer the consumer to adopt less costly lifestyle behaviors.

Risk Rating

One such incentive is risk-rated insurance premiums. Most simply this means that those whose voluntarily chosen lifestyle behaviors are shown to lead to excess health care costs pay higher premiums to offset those increased costs. These costs are now well understood and quantified (Anderson, Haight, Jose, & Brink, 1989; Anderson & Jose, 1987a, 1987b; Bertera, 1990; Bly, Jones, & Richardson, 1986; Brink, 1987; Erfurt, Foote, & Heirich, 1991; Jones, Bly, & Richardson, 1990; Jose & Anderson, 1986, 1988,

1991; Jose, Anderson, & Haight, 1987; Opatz, 1987; Vickery, Golaszewski, Wright, & McPhee, 1986).

Innovative companies are now taking the lead in structuring programs that provide a more equitable basis on which to determine health care premium contributions (A. Foster Higgins & Co., 1990; New York Business Group on Health, 1990). These are pioneering efforts, and many suffer from problems associated with a new and emerging technology that is trying to provide incentives for healthy lifestyles at the workplace (Washington Business Group on Health, 1992). There are many issues in plan design and implementation that are critical to both the effectiveness of the plan and its ethical responsibility. These issues are addressed later in this chapter.

Fundamental to the concept of risk rating is a new quid pro quo in the employer-employee contract regarding health insurance. The reality is that the employer can no longer cover all health- and illness-related expenses of employees and spouses. The employer must require—and the employee must recognize this requirement to be just—that employees take reasonably good care of what their company is insuring. This is currently the case with regard to equipment and machinery that an employer provides for the use for employees at the worksite. For example, employees are expected to take reasonably good care of the capital equipment they use, such as typewriters, computers, and production machinery. Similarly, employers may require in the future that employees take reasonably good care of the human capital that is insured by the company by conscientiously attending their own and their families' health habits.

Cost of Risks

There should no longer be any doubt that lifestyle choices made by employees significantly affect organizational health care costs. Since 1979, the U.S. Surgeon General has issued a series of reports on the consequences of behavioral health risks (Dept. of Health, Education, and Welfare, 1979; Dept. of Health & Human Services, 1980, 1986, 1988a, 1988b, 1991). The cost of behavioral health risks is well known. The excess health care costs of those who have poor lifestyle habits can amount to thousands of dollars a person a year (Anderson, Haight, Jose, & Brink, 1989; Bertera, 1990; Brink, 1987). These are costs that would not have been incurred if employees practiced healthful lifestyle habits. These excess costs appear in many forms: increased utilization of health care services, premature death, increased disability, increased workers' compensation claims, increased worker replacement costs, increased sick leave, and lowered productivity.

A definitive study on the issue of the relationship between lifestyle risks and health care costs (Brink, 1987) was also reported in the *Wall Street Journal* ("Study lays groundwork," 1987). This study, based on a

40,000-person-year data base, highlighted the differences in health care costs for those at high, moderate, and low risk. For example, those who smoke have 18% higher medical claims and are 43% more likely than nonsmokers to miss 1 week of work each year. Sedentary employees spend 30% more days in the hospital and are 20% more likely than active individuals to call in sick more than 7 days a year. Seriously overweight workers are 48% more likely to have claims exceeding $5,000 in 1 year and 29% more likely to miss more than 1 week of work a year, compared to workers nearer their ideal body weights.

Similarly, there can no longer be any serious doubt concerning the effectiveness of health promotion programs in slowing the escalation of organizational health care costs. Many researchers have demonstrated organizational cost savings due to lifestyle risk reduction programs (Anderson & Jose, 1987a, 1987b; Anderson et al., 1989; Bertera, 1990; Bly et al., 1986; Erfurt et al., 1991; Jones et al., 1990; Jose & Anderson, 1991; Jose et al., 1987; Opatz, 1987; Vickery et al., 1986).

The risk-rated approach to health insurance premiums has two simple goals: To make more equitable the basis on which health insurance premiums are determined, and to motivate individuals to lower their lifestyle-related health risks. Some argue that this approach displays an inappropriate paternalism on the part of employers or insurers, or that risk rating is inappropriate for other reasons, including the argument that it is discriminatory under the Americans With Disabilities Act (Frierson, 1992; New York Business Group on Health, 1990; Terry, 1991). As with any new program, there are unanswered questions about risk rating. Companies will have to review the issues for themselves in light of their own needs, those of their employees, and the corporate culture to decide whether risk rating is appropriate and if so, how it should be implemented. Indeed, employees have a legitimate complaint if employers or insurers are overly paternalistic. However, the issue at stake here is not paternalism, but rather corporate business strategy, competitive advantage in the marketplace, and equity for employees in the face of rapidly rising health care expenditures. Offering incentives to employees to lower their risk levels and consequently reduce their need for health care services does not indicate paternalism, but a recognition of the economic realities of the health care situation in modern business. A company that can reduce its health care expenses, the most rapidly growing cost to many businesses, is one that will gain a competitive advantage.

Principles of Risk Rating

Fundamental to the concept of risk rating as a motivational tool is the realization that the organizations in which we spend our working lives have a profound impact on our attitudes and behavior by overtly and covertly communicating expectations and standards for acceptable behaviors. Many of these behaviors are relevant to the reduction or increase in health risks. If, for instance your coworkers are of the "burgers-and-beer" crowd, you will find it difficult to maintain healthful eating habits when socializing with them or trying to "fit in."

Organizational Policies and Programs

Organizations have great power to influence employee behaviors through organizational policies and programs. Personnel policies set standards of acceptable or desired employee behavior. Company "perks," awards, and recognitions also set standards by which the organization judges employee behavior and job excellence.

Organizations now use these instruments more consciously to address employee attitudes and behaviors in the area of health practices. Policies on alcohol consumption and seat belt use while on the job are specific examples of common corporate policies that deal with lifestyle behaviors. Management actions that can have a impact on employee behavior include

- a written commitment to a healthy work force,
- a comprehensive health promotion program,
- supportive organizational policies, and
- supportive benefit programs, *including* risk-rated health insurance.

More companies are coming to view the establishment of health promotion programs and risk-rated insurance premiums as an extension of this concept of establishing standards and expectations for employees relevant to healthful practices. Companies are increasingly willing to think in these terms in part because they are beginning to see health promotion not as an employee benefit but as a core business strategy for containing health care costs. It is now possible to estimate the excess costs, or liability, associated with behavioral health risks in the employee population. Also, executives can model the effects of a company program on risk reduction and make long-term projections regarding possible return on their financial investment. Thus, executives can make decisions about investment in health promotion and risk rating on the same basis that they make investment decisions in other areas of business. With its potential for controlling health care costs and creating a healthier, more productive work force, risk rating seems more and more compelling to many corporate leaders.

Success Factors

The promise of investment in health promotion and risk rating can fail in two ways. It may fail to reduce overall organizational risk, or it may fail to be cost effective. However, a well-designed program maximizes the likelihood of success on both criteria. There are inherent difficulties in designing effective and cost-effective programs, but there also are some basic principles that can guide the process. Of course, specific details must be tailored to the organization's culture and operating style. The challenge to benefit plan managers is to

- establish innovative leadership,
- assure positive return on investment, and
- be ethically responsible.

More than anything else, innovative leadership is required, not only to address the problem of escalating health care costs in general, but to address specifically the issues concerning risk-rated insurance plans. The basic approach is really quite simple. The plan must link good health habits to reduced employee cost for plan participation and encourage appropriate use of preventive services. This second point is often overlooked, but it is extremely important if an organization is to reduce health care costs.

Assuring a return on investment is not easy. However, it is possible to make decisions and structure plans so that this is the likely outcome. This requires both a well-structured plan and a financial analysis that aids in identifying and quantifying the relevant costs and benefits.

Four Principles of Plan Design

There are four principles that can help guide the development and implementation of health promotion and risk-rated incentive plans.

- Provide a financial incentive for employees to do the "right things."
- Structure the program to assure a positive return on investment.
- Preserve equity.
- Maintain the organization's ethical responsibility.

The "right things" are fairly simple: They include exercising regularly, eating a diet low in fat, cholesterol, salt, and sugar and high in grains, legumes, and carbohydrates, and giving up smoking. These practices result in increased cardiac endurance and lower percent body fat, blood cholesterol levels, and blood pressure. These in turn lead to a decrease in morbidity and premature mortality in the work force. The "right" list could also include other factors, such as wearing seat belts and learning to manage on-the-job stress; but the first principle behind any risk-rated health insurance plan is to provide a monetary incentive for employees who achieve acceptable levels of risk on each of the measured risk factors.

The case study of Foldcraft Corporation presented in this chapter illustrates one company's approach.

Structuring the program to assure a positive return on investment requires estimating the net of program costs and benefits over a period of time. Reallocating already budgeted organizational costs rather than incurring new costs for program implementation can make this easier. For example, if an organization has budgeted 6% for salary increases in the coming year, 1% of that increase could be distributed through a risk-rated insurance incentive plan. This idea makes sense, because it rewards those employees whose behaviors are consistent with core business strategies. Sales and marketing personnel, for example, are typically compensated under a plan with similar logic. Creating an investment in this way does not require a new funding source.

Another strategy for helping assure a positive return is to structure the plan so that there is no net cost to the organization. This can be accomplished by lowering insurance rates for low-risk employees while raising rates for high-risk employees. For example, if an organization knows both what its total insurance premium will be and what the incentive structure of the risk-rated program is, rates can be set so that the combination of lower rates for low-risk employees and higher rates for high-risk employees generates the same total insurance premium as the organization's previous plan. This is probably best done at the time of insurance renewal when rate adjustments are expected.

These examples are not exhaustive, but they illustrate the point that it is possible to design plan components that will optimize a company's potential return on its investment.

The third principle, preserve equity, is essential for employee acceptance of a plan. Some organizations have mistakenly implemented programs that have violated this principle by rewarding only those who *reduce* risks, while ignoring those who are already at low risk. A good example is the company that pays smokers $200 if they quit smoking. Long-term employees who have never smoked are rightfully indignant that their contribution to lowering health care costs over the years is not being recognized or rewarded appropriately. In fact, this could encourage nonsmokers to take up the habit so they can qualify for the incentive to quit! Any program design must consider carefully the impact of equity issues.

No company should knowingly violate the last principle of plan design: Maintain the organization's ethical responsibility. Many have done it unwittingly, however. In the process of structuring incentives, an organization is, in a sense, inviting its employees to play a game in which, if they are clever, they can earn the incentive. Employees for the most part are rather clever. Therefore, they will seek out the most efficient way to earn the rewards. This is exactly what the organization desires, that is, it desires to influence the behavior of its employees.

The problem arises when clever employees devise strategies that management had not anticipated and that are counterproductive to the organizational goals. An example is the company that offers a reward each month to work groups that have had no down-time injuries. The incentive is intended to cultivate an environment in which employees are careful, help each other avoid injury, and use safety equipment and procedures. It may also produce a system in which employees cover for an injured worker who needs immediate attention. In the long run, both the employer and the employee may pay more for delayed health care services, disability, and lost productivity.

Key Issues in Plan Design

One key issue in plan design is the use of reward instead of punishment. Behavioral research has demonstrated that reward is generally more effective than punishment in evoking desired behaviors. Therefore, whenever possible the incentives and the risk-rating structures should be designed to *reward* desired behavior rather than to punish undesired behavior. Furthermore, the program should include various levels of desired behavior with incremental rewards; as employees more closely conform to the desired behavior standard, they receive higher rewards.

Because they typically account for more than half of an organization's health care costs, involving dependents in the program is important. Spouses, too, should be encouraged to participate in health risk appraisals, health screenings, and risk reduction components of the program. It may even be reasonable to *require* spousal participation and then average employee and spouse risk levels to determine the overall incentive level of the employee.

Designing a plan that incorporates these considerations and tailoring it to a specific organization's constraints, values, and culture is an intricate and demanding task. The following case study illustrates how one company resolved these issues while implementing an innovative, risk-based insurance incentive system.

Risk Rating in Practice—The Foldcraft Corporation

In 1989 Foldcraft Corporation was feeling the pain—the pain of rising health care costs. The founder and chairman of the board had made the decision in 1983 to "hold the line" on company contributions to increasing health care costs. For several years, increases were passed on to employees, which caused widespread dissatisfaction with the health care benefits plan. The plan became so expensive that many considered it a negative benefit. Employees were leaving the company plan to seek their own insurance or were going without insurance. By August 1989, only 47% of employees were enrolled in the company plan (Foldcraft corporate records). Not only did this shrink the risk base for the company plan, it also made it more difficult to shop for alternative insurance carriers.

The director of human resources was in a quandary. He was under pressure to provide rate relief for employees, but he could see no real solution to the problem of escalating health care costs. The only way out was to reduce demand for health care. This, the company decided, meant providing behavioral health risk screening and health risk assessment in conjunction with a risk-rated financial incentive for employees to lower risks.

Company Background

Foldcraft is a 300-employee, nonunion company that manufactures restaurant and public seating—booths, tables, and chairs. The company is a solely owned corporation with operations of about $20 million a year. Foldcraft is located in a single facility in Kenyon, Minnesota, a rural community of 1,500 people in the center of an agricultural area. Foldcraft also has an employee stock ownership plan (ESOP); 49% of the company is owned by its employees.

Foldcraft had a nascent health promotion program, which began in 1982. It consisted of informal exercise groups, luncheon group meetings, and a point-based exercise program in which participants could earn $15 to $25 a week. This program did not gain widespread acceptance by employees and did not attract those who most needed it because it was primarily exercise-based, it was not integrated into the strategic goals of the company, and employees did not view participation in the program as an important corporate objective. However, perhaps most significantly because it set a precedent, Foldcraft had instituted a program of no smoking within company buildings and at that time had a policy of not hiring smokers.

The company recognized, however, that health promotion could be an effective force in reducing employee risks, increasing productivity, and slowing the escalation of health care costs. In summer 1989, after attending the annual National Wellness Association meeting, the director of human resources and I began to discuss the option of implementing a risk-rated health insurance plan at Foldcraft.

Program Description

Our discussions identified five plan objectives.

1. Provide health insurance rate relief for employees.

2. Increase the number of employees participating in the insurance plan.
3. Reduce employee health risks.
4. Lower long-term insurance rate increases.
5. Collect current corporate risk data to provide a baseline for assessing change.

To accomplish these objectives, we devised a plan with two distinct incentive features: a participation incentive and a healthy lifestyle incentive. The primary objectives addressed by the participation incentive were 1, 2, and 5: to provide rate relief, to increase plan participation by lowering the cost, and to determine the corporate risk baseline. To earn the participation incentive, both employee and spouse (if covered by the plan) were required to participate in the health risk appraisal and screening process. All employees were eligible to participate in the health risk appraisal and screening, but only those on the company health plan were eligible for the incentives. Employees were required to be rescreened annually to maintain their program eligibility.

The health risk appraisal used was "HealthPath," which is available through StayWell Health Management Systems, Inc., Eagan, Minnesota. The screening process included specific physiological tests related to six risk factors:

- Tobacco use (saliva thiocyanate)
- Percent body fat (impedance method)
- Blood pressure (standard cuff)
- Total cholesterol (finger stick, Reflotron)
- Oxygen uptake (step test)
- Flexibility (sit-and-reach test)

There were two incentives for participation in this portion of the program. First, all participating employees received 1-1/2 hours paid time-off to participate in the screening and the interpretation session. Second, each employee who participated in the company-sponsored health care plan received an additional premium contribution from the company of $20 a month. This amounted to an extra $240 a year in take-home pay.

The second incentive feature of the program, the healthy lifestyle incentive, addresses plan objectives 2, 3, and 4: increase plan participation by reducing the cost, motivate employees to lower their health risks, and slow the upward trend in health care costs. The idea of the healthy lifestyle incentive is to create different health care premium rates based on the degree of risk an employee chooses. In this program, only the employees' risk levels are taken into account when determining their risk rating, not the spouses' risk levels. However, an aggregate rating of both employee's and spouse's risks appears to be a good idea and may be included in a future revision of the plan.

The goal was to create an overall rating of an employee's risks that would reflect the extent to which that individual could be expected, on average, to exceed the health care costs of an individual with no behavioral health risks. To do this, an employee is given a risk level from 1 to 5 on each of six measured risks. The numerical risk on each risk factor is then multiplied by a weighting factor that indicates the relative contribution of that risk factor to health care costs. (The weighting factors used were developed from a proprietary risk analysis system.) This produces a weighted risk level for each measured risk. These weighted risk levels are then summed across all six risks to produce a composite risk score. The composite risk score is then converted to one of five composite risk levels. Each of the five composite risk levels represents a different overall behavioral risk level and is tied to a corresponding premium contribution from the company. The lower the overall risk level, the higher the company contribution. Like the participation incentive, this premium is also paid monthly and is seen as an increase in take-home pay.

The premium contribution at each composite risk level is shown in Table 8.1. The contribution for the very low risk category was set so that, when combined with the participation incentive, the full cost of health care for the single individual would be covered. The total premium contribution under this plan is calculated by adding the participation incentive ($20 a month) and the healthy lifestyle incentive.

The participation incentive is a feature that was designed to meet a specific need at Foldcraft and should not be mistaken as an essential feature of a risk-rated plan. Generally speaking, a separate incentive specifically for participation is ill-advised. The guiding principle of a risk-rated insurance plan should be to provide incentives only for demonstrated low behavioral-risk levels.

Table 8.1
Healthy Lifestyle Premium Contribution

Overall risk level	Participation incentive	Healthy lifestyle incentive	Total premium contribution
Very low risk	$20/mo = $240/yr	$40/mo = $480/yr	$60/mo = $720/yr
Low risk	$20/mo = $240/yr	$30/mo = $360/yr	$50/mo = $600/yr
Average risk	$20/mo = $240/yr	$20/mo = $240/yr	$40/mo = $480/yr
High risk	$20/mo = $240/yr	$5/mo = $60/yr	$25/mo = $300/yr
Very high risk	$20/mo = $240/yr	$0/mo = $0/yr	$20/mo = $240/yr

Implementation Process

The new plan was first presented to Foldcraft's executive team in October 1989. It was approved, and the program was announced 2 weeks later. Implementation of the screening component was scheduled for November, and risk-adjusted premiums went into effect in January 1990. At the program announcement, the rationale underlying the company's commitment to the program was explained. Escalating health care costs were a major threat to the company. Healthier employees, besides using fewer health care resources, were more productive, absent from work less often, and generally had a more optimistic outlook on life. It was also explained that program participation would be voluntary and could only help, not hurt, an employee from a financial point of view. Confidentiality of all information collected was also stressed.

The screening was conducted on-site for each of the two shifts by the SHAPE program of the Park Nicollet Medical Foundation, based in Minneapolis. An experienced team provided a professional yet informal atmosphere, which inspired employee trust and confidence. Screening was done on company time and at company expense; no copayments or fees of any kind were involved. The screening was available to all employees and spouses, whether they were on the company-sponsored health plan or not, and arrangements were made to screen working spouses at their convenience.

After screening, an individual results booklet was prepared and presented to each participant in the context of group interpretation sessions. These sessions were also free to employees and spouses and were provided on company time.

Company executives participated in the screening along with other employees. Even the 70-year-old founder and chairman of the board and his wife participated. This demonstration of executive commitment to the program was probably the key to the high participation rate achieved in this first screening (82% of employees, according to Foldcraft records).

After the interpretation sessions, employees who wished to participate in the incentive portion of the plan turned in their risk scores to the plan administrator for calculation of their new premiums. Individual risk scores reached the plan administrator only through this route. Providing risk information to the company remained totally within the control of the individual employee. Employees who wanted to qualify for a lower risk status were scheduled for follow-up screenings. The first of these was held in February 1990.

Reactions to the Program

Employee reaction was tentative at first, due to concerns about confidentiality, the screening process, and general uncertainty about just how the new plan would affect them. The potential savings on premiums, however, was large enough to raise considerable interest in the program.

Employee reaction became more positive on the first screening day due to the professional and friendly demeanor of the screening staff. As screened employees related their experiences to coworkers, interest and participation soared.

Executive employees also participated. In fact virtually every executive employee took some significant personal step toward increased fitness. For example, some purchased exercise equipment for their private use—one bought a rowing machine, another a stationary bicycle, another a treadmill. After these commitments on the part of executives helped employees understand that this was not just a human relations program, but a core component of the Foldcraft business strategy, attendance at weekly wellness meetings rose 50%. Attendance at guest presentations on wellness topics also increased.

The initial wariness displayed by employees largely disappeared, because the company demonstrated its concern for individual privacy and confidentiality of data. Today there appears to be no fear or nervousness on the part of employees regarding the program. In the short time the program has existed, it has become part of the corporate culture, the normal way of doing business at Foldcraft.

The reaction to this program from other businesses has been overwhelming. Our presentations at national and regional meetings have elicited queries from every part of the country and from all types and sizes of organizations. Newsletters, magazines, and newspapers serving the wellness, human resources, and benefits communities have picked up on our risk-rating concepts and spread the news throughout their constituencies.

Preliminary Indicators of Success

There are a number of indications, both formal and informal, of the success of our program. Informal indicators include those observations, which were not originally part of the evaluation plan, regarding the attitudes, values, and behaviors of company employees. Formal indicators are defined by the formal evaluation plan, which assesses the program's effectiveness relative to its original five objectives.

The informal, often serendipitous, success indicators are in some ways the most significant because they reveal the extent to which the organizational culture has been influenced by the program. Our favorite is what we have called the "donut index." A long-standing Foldcraft tradition was that for each injury-free workweek, the company would provide free sweet rolls for the next Wednesday's morning break. In the interest of employee health, fresh fruit was added to the offering. After the incentive program began, so many donuts were left over each week that the order had to be reduced until it stabilized at about half of what it had been. On the other hand, the "fruit index" has risen. So now instead of a donut break, Foldcraft takes a fruit break.

The participation of top officers of the company has already been mentioned. We have called this the "executive action index." Their example, while not systematically measured, has been an important influence in modifying the corporate culture.

Coinciding with program initiation, a health coordinator was hired to oversee health promotion programming. Interest among employees was so great that she was overwhelmed by requests for assistance.

Foldcraft has an interesting voluntary drug screening program. Those who sign up are screened on a random basis. Consistent with the new health orientation of the employees, approximately 90% of employees have signed up for the program, including executive team members.

A fifth informal success indicator is the interest that has been generated from other companies around the country. Interest has been so great that responding to it has become a serious drain on the human resources department. Yet each inquiry receives attention, not only to share the Foldcraft experience, but also to learn what other organizations are doing.

Formal success indicators are geared toward quantitative evaluation of the five program objectives. A written evaluation program is in place. Although it will be several years before conclusive results are available, the initial indicators are encouraging. Our efforts to obtain a reliable company-risk baseline (Objective 5) was very successful, with 82% of employees participating in the health risk appraisal and screening. Clearly the program has been effective in providing rate relief for employees (Objective 1), particularly for low-risk employees. Insurance plan participation also seems to be increasing (Objective 2). In 2 months, overall employee participation increased 10%, from 47% to 57% (Foldcraft program evaluation). New hire enrollment over the same period increased 15%, from 35% to 50% (Foldcraft program evaluation). These indicators are encouraging, but it will be several years before the other two objectives, risk reduction (Objective 3) and health care cost containment (Objective 4), can be evaluated.

Summary

As with any new or innovative human resources program, there are still many unresolved issues related to risk-rating health insurance premiums based on behavioral health risks. I have identified the key issues and outlined a specific program that has been implemented to address them.

I argue that risk-rated health insurance offers an equitable way to distribute the costs of individual insurance premiums and that it offers the company another strategy for dealing with the long-term escalation in health care costs.

There are still many unanswered questions: legal, ethical, financial, and scientific. As more is learned about these issues, risk-rated programs will need to be modified appropriately. At this time, however, it is fair to conclude that such programs can be designed and implemented in a way that averts the most prevalent fears regarding employee morale and legal concerns. In fact, this type of program can be an extremely positive one both for employees and for the organization.

References

A. Foster Higgins & Co. (1990). Integration of wellness initiatives and financial incentives in employer sponsored benefit plans. Washington, DC: Author.

Anderson, D.R., Haight, S.A., Jose, W.S., & Brink, S.R. (1989, July). *Lifestyle and medical costs: Multivariate models linking health risks and health care claims*. Paper presented at the National Wellness Conference, Stevens Point, WI.

Anderson, D.R., & Jose, W.S. (1987a). Employee lifestyle and the bottom line: Results from the StayWell evaluation. *Fitness in Business, 2*, 86-91.

Anderson, D.R., & Jose, W.S. (1987b). Comprehensive evaluation of a worksite health promotion program: The StayWell program at Control Data. In S.H. Klarreich (Ed.), *Health and fitness in the workplace: Health education in business organizations* (pp. 284-289). New York: Praeger.

Bertera, R.L. (1990). The effects of workplace health promotion on absenteeism and employment costs in a large industrial population. *American Journal of Public Health, 80*(9), 1101-1105.

Bly, J.L., Jones, R.C., & Richardson, J.E. (1986). Impact of worksite health promotion on health care costs and utilization. *Journal of the American Medical Association, 256*, 3235-3240.

Brink, S.D. (1987). *Health risks and behavior: The impact on medical costs*. Milwaukee: Milliman & Robertson.

Department of Health, Education, & Welfare. (1979). *Report on health promotion and disease prevention: Healthy people* (DHEW Publication No. 79-055071). Washington, DC: U.S. Government Printing Office.

Department of Health & Human Services. (1980). *Promoting health/preventing disease: Objectives for the nation* (DHHS Publication No. 455-321-20079). Washington, DC: U.S. Government Printing Office.

Department of Health & Human Services. (1986). *The 1990 health objectives for the nation: A midcourse review* (DHHS Publication No. 191-691-70228). Washington, DC: U.S. Government Printing Office.

Department of Health & Human Services. (1988a). *The health consequences of smoking: Nicotine addiction—A report of the Surgeon General* (DHHS Publication No. 88-8406). Washington, DC: U.S. Government Printing Office.

Department of Health & Human Services. (1988b). *The Surgeon General's report on nutrition and health* (DHHS Publication No. 017-001-004-65-1). Washington, DC: U.S. Government Printing Office.

Department of Health & Human Services. (1991). *Healthy people 2000: National health promotion and disease prevention objectives* (DHHS Publication No. 91-50212). Washington, DC: U.S. Government Printing Office.

Erfurt, J.C., Foote, A., & Heirich, M.A. (1991). Worksite wellness programs: Incremental comparison of screening and referral alone, health education, follow-up counseling, and plant organization. *American Journal of Health Promotion*, **5**(6), 438-448.

Frierson, J.C. (1992, May-June). New laws may make employee health incentive plans illegal. *Journal of Compensation and Benefits*, pp. 5-9.

Jones, R.C., Bly, J.L., & Richardson, J.E. (1990). A study of worksite health promotion and absenteeism: Evaluation of the LIVE FOR LIFE program. *Journal of Occupational Medicine*, **32**, 95-99.

Jose, W.S., & Anderson, D.R. (1986). Control Data: The StayWell program. *Corporate Commentary*, **2**, 1-13.

Jose, W.S., & Anderson, D.R. (1988). Paying the price for unhealthy workers. *Healthy Companies*, **1**, 3.

Jose, W.S., & Anderson, D.R. (1991). Control Data's StayWell program: A health cost management strategy. In S.M. Weiss, J. E. Fielding, & A. Baum (Eds.), *Perspectives in behavioral medicine: Health at work* (pp. 49-72). Hillsdale, NJ: Erlbaum.

Jose, W.S., Anderson, D.R., & Haight, S.A. (1987). The StayWell strategy for health care cost containment. In J.P. Opatz (Ed.), *Health promotion evaluation: Measuring the organizational impact* (pp. 15-34). Stevens Point, WI: National Wellness Institute.

New York Business Group on Health, Inc. Discussion Paper (1990, May). Risk-rated health insurance: Incentives for healthy lifestyles. **10**(1), 1-2.

Opatz, J.P. (Ed.) (1987). *Health promotion evaluation: Measuring the organizational impact*. Stevens Point, WI: National Wellness Institute.

Study lays groundwork for tying health care costs to worker's behavior. (1987, April 14). *The Wall Street Journal*, p. 35.

Terry, P.E. (1991, February). Of risk and reason—the battle over risk rating: A dangerous innovation. *Health Action Managers*, pp. 1, 6-9.

Vickery, D.M., Golaszewski, T., Wright, E., & McPhee, L.E. (1986). Lifestyle and organizational health insurance costs. *Journal of Occupational Medicine, 28,* 1165-1168.

Washington Business Group on Health. (1992). *The challenge of financial incentives and risk rating: A collection of essays and case studies.* Washington, DC: Author.

Chapter 9

Medical Benefits Cost Containment: The Municipal Government of Birmingham, Alabama

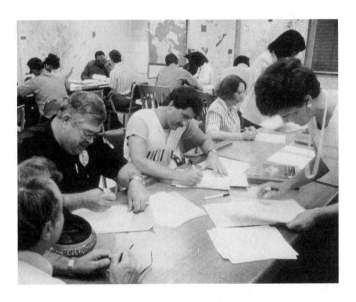

R. William Whitmer
James C. Hilyer
Kathleen C. Brown

Current and projected costs of medical benefits are a major concern for the chief executive, financial officers, and personnel directors of most corporations and governments. A recent survey pointed out that 63% of CEOs feel that medical benefit expenses are the #1 short- and long-term corporate concern, and 83% considered it one of the top three concerns (Issues & Trends, 1992). Such expenses are also a source of frustration.

When CEOs and CFOs were surveyed as a single group, 86% said they feel they have little or no direct control in containing or reducing the cost of medical benefits (News Briefs, 1991).

Medical benefits expenses are eroding net profits or reserves at an alarming rate. In 1965, these expenses amounted to about 7% of net profits in the average company. In 1991, 42% of companies reported that medical benefits amounted to 30% or more of net profits. Further analysis of this group indicates that 24% said medical expenses were more than 50% of net profits, and 14% reported that medical expenses exceeded 75% of net profits (Data Watch, 1992).

Because of the rapid and seemingly uncontrolled rise in medical benefits expenses, executives from both the private and public sectors are interested in solutions that may moderate increases or actually decrease costs. One proposed solution is worksite wellness or health promotion programs. Managers understand preventive maintenance for machinery and hardware. They not only expect but require that machinery be lubricated, bearings replaced, electrical circuits rewired, and everything kept clean in order to extend operational longevity. Few managers, however, emotionally or intellectually apply this same principle to employees. This may be due to lack of information or understanding, given that the medical profession states that 50% to 60% of all diseases and medical problems, both physical and mental, are preventable (Castelli, 1992). The other reason for the lack of widespread acceptance of employee health promotion is the lack of reliable, reproducible data that prove the effectiveness of worksite health promotion programs in reducing the cost of medical benefits.

Although health promotion is increasing in popularity as a cost-containment tool, other potentially effective efforts have probably been used more frequently, namely, medical plan redesign including cost shifting and managed care. We report in this chapter on the findings of a cost-containment project conducted for the employees of the municipal government of Birmingham, Alabama, that emphasized health promotion and also included managed care and plan redesign.

Characteristics of a Municipal Government

When considering data from the public sector, the question should be raised, can the health promotion experiences of a municipal government be extrapolated to the private sector? The answer is yes. Though there may be certain logistical differences between private and public sector employee groups, generally employees, program needs, and responses are similar.

The city government has 30 separate departments. The largest departments are police, fire and rescue, and streets and sanitation. Other major departments include traffic engineering, libraries, the zoo, the airport, the museums, the civic center, civil defense, building inspections, and parks and recreation. Administrative departments include the mayor's office, personnel, finance, legal, and the city council. This mixture creates a complex challenge when attempting to produce health promotion programs. Work hours vary from the traditional 8 to 5 shift to the fire and rescue schedule of 24 hours on duty and the next 48 hours off. The police department works three shifts around the clock.

Another major challenge in working with a city employee population is the diversity in educational and socioeconomic backgrounds. Approximately 60% of all employees are blue-collar workers, 50% are members of minority groups, and 20% are female.

The City of Birmingham's Cost-Containment Program

To study the medical effectiveness and cost-effectiveness of worksite health promotion programs, along with other cost-containment efforts, a controlled experimental health promotion program was designed and implemented for the employees and selected dependents of the municipal government of the city of Birmingham. This study, which was conducted from 1985 through 1990, was funded jointly by the National Institutes of Health (NIH), the National Heart, Lung and Blood Institute, and by the city of Birmingham.

Birmingham has a population of 266,000. It is totally surrounded by several independent cities, which together create a greater metropolitan area with a population of about 1 million (Bureau of the Census, 1990). The city had 3,586 full-time employees in 1985 and 4,000 employees in 1990. The employee population, therefore, grew by about 2% a year during the project period (Personnel Dept., 1991). City employees work at over 100 different worksites, which are spread over 154 square miles. Many do not have a fixed work station, such as a desk or a production location.

There are several unions operating within the city government. In establishing the city health promotion program, and during its operation, efforts were made to solicit union cooperation and support and to counter any negative impressions.

Why Birmingham Started Its Program

For the 9-year period prior to the study, medical benefits expenses increased at a rate nearly twice the national average (Feasibility Study,

1984). As shown in Figure 9.1, during these years, medical benefits costs increased from $1.5 million to $7.6 million. Medical expenses increased from 16% to 40% of total benefits and from 3.8% to 11.6% of total payroll.

From 1974 to 1983, the city had a traditional insurance plan that was experience-rated. City officials calculated that if the trend observed during these years continued, the cost of medical benefits would be $33 million in 1990. Projected increases of this magnitude were judged unacceptable.

Feasibility Study Recommendations

As the beginning of a cost-management program, a large medical benefits consulting firm was hired to conduct a feasibility study and make recommendations for cost containment. The firm offered these suggestions.

1. Discontinue the traditional insurance coverage plan and begin a self-insured, self-administered plan.
2. Redesign the medical benefits plan to include no copayment for office visits, second opinions, utilization review, preadmission certification, and other cost-containment strategies.
3. Build and staff a comprehensive fitness center for the use of city employees.

Finally, even though it was not among the feasibility study recommendations, about 6 months after the start of the self-insured indemnity plan, the first health maintenance organization (HMO) became available and was offered as an alternative to the indemnity plan.

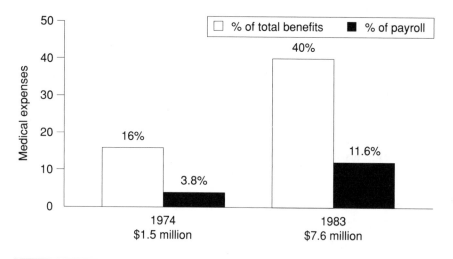

Figure 9.1 Medical benefits expenses for Birmingham city employees for 1974 and 1983. *Note.* Data from Personnel Department, City of Birmingham, AL.

Program Design and Methodology

Another recommendation of the feasibility study was to provide an employee wellness program. The funding for an initial, small-scale, pilot project came from first-year savings when the city converted to a self-insured, self-administered medical benefits plan. Funding for the 1-year pilot wellness program amounted to $200,000. The wellness program was designed, developed, marketed, and produced through a joint venture between Wellness South, Inc., a private health promotion consulting firm, and the University of Alabama at Birmingham (UAB) Medical Center, Division of General and Preventive Medicine.

Marketing activities included a slide presentation for all employees who attended small group meetings. Immediately following the presentation, 83% of the employees volunteered for the wellness program. Of the 2,986 volunteers, 1,100 were randomly selected and divided into two groups, a wellness group of 550 and a control group of equal size. All 1,100 completed a health risk appraisal and participated in a medical screening. The medical screening recorded family and personal history, resting and exercise heart rate, blood pressure, weight, height, percent body fat, cholesterol, HDL cholesterol, cardiac risk index, triglycerides, blood glucose, and hematocrit.

Following the medical screening, all employees in the wellness group were encouraged to attend a health information session (HIS) every 2 weeks during work hours. HIS's were 50-minute, self-contained presentations on topics such as how to write a personal exercise prescription, reading food labels, AIDS, sleep disorders, how to select a physician, and how to prevent back injury.

Attendance at HIS's ranged from 441 (out of 550) to 86. The low-attendance programs were targeted to specific health topics, such as arthritis and sleep disturbances, and were not expected to attract as many participants as topics like nutrition or fitness. In all, there were 4,294 employee-hours of exposure to health-related information.

The wellness group also attended comprehensive intervention programs, including smoking cessation, weight reduction, stress management, hypertension control, and cholesterol modification. These classes met weekly for 5 to 12 weeks, depending on the topic. Intervention programs were conducted immediately after working hours. The HISs and intervention programs were presented at city hall, fire stations, police precincts, and other work locations. Employees in the control group did not have access to intervention programs or HISs.

A total of 260 employees, or nearly one half the wellness group, participated in the intervention programs. Forty-three percent participated in weight-reduction programs, 18% in smoking cessation, 16% in stress management, 13% in cholesterol modification, and 10% in hypertension control. An estimated 130 additional employees wanted to enroll in intervention programs before the pilot project ended.

Follow-up studies of those who participated in the weight-reduction programs indicated 76% with weight losses between 5 and 100 pounds. Of those attending smoking cessation programs, 55% had stopped smoking at the end of 6 months.

Based on the 1984 to 1985 pilot program experience, the decision was made to respond to a request for proposal from NIH for a worksite health promotion program grant.

The NIH Program

The grant application was generated by and awarded to the university. The grant was in the amount of $1.5 million, with matching funds provided by the city. The $3 million budget allowed the limited pilot program to be expanded and offered to all employees for at least 5 years of continuous operation. NIH rated the application favorably because the city already had a functioning wellness program that included many blue-collar and minority workers. Matching funds from the city were also a factor.

The basic project design included an annual medical screening each year for 5 consecutive years, aggressive physician referral, and various health education and intervention programs. The medical screening included personal and family medical history, height, weight, fitness testing, percent body fat, blood pressure, spirometry, cholesterol, HDL-cholesterol, triglyceride, blood glucose and hematocrit measurements, and calculation of a cardiac risk index. The screening was conducted at one of the municipal auditoriums. Employees were permitted to travel to the location during work hours. The medical screenings were conducted by personnel from the university and from Wellness South. Selected employees who were certified paramedics from the fire and rescue service assisted by drawing blood and conducting other testing procedures. A physician was on-site at all times.

Medical Screen Participation

When medical screens are voluntary, those who decline to participate often are those who exhibit multiple risk factors (Jones, Samkoff, Wolff, & Bowers, 1991). Because only a small number of employees utilize the major portion of medical benefit dollars (Edington, 1992), employees who decline to participate may represent those multiple-risk employees. Participation by *all* employees is essential in order to obtain an unbiased estimate of program effectiveness. Therefore, the project directors wanted to avoid problems associated with voluntary participation.

A thorough review of the literature yielded no example of a large health promotion program in which all employees had participated in a medical screening. It was felt that not only was it important to program evaluation for all employees to participate in the medical screen, but it would also be a "first" in health promotion. In response, the city sought expert legal opinion that suggested the medical screen could be made a part of the medical benefits plan if written in as such. Consequently, the plan was rewritten, and participation in the annual medical screen was made a prerequisite for medical benefits. Employees were not required to participate, but if they declined, they would not have access to the medical benefits plan. On the average, annual participation in the medical screen from 1985 through 1990 was approximately 95% of full-time employees.

Since the medical screen was a stated prerequisite for medical benefits, it was necessary for all medical data to be completely confidential. The employer received no medical data information about individual employees. Results of medical screening were mailed in a confidential envelope to each employee's home, and a copy was sent to the employee's personal physician if requested by the employee.

Program Protocol

Birmingham's project was designed to evaluate medical effectiveness and cost-effectiveness. Because participation and health outcome data are still being analyzed, this chapter focuses on cost-effectiveness, which had an extraordinary outcome. The other data will be the subject of future publications, but the basic protocol gives an idea of the magnitude of the city's effort.

After the medical screen, employees were randomly assigned to one of four equally sized groups:

- Group A—Had access to all segments of the program at no cost. Members could attend any desired intervention programs. All services and programs were available to spouses at no charge.
- Group B—Same as Group A, except spouses could not participate.
- Group C—Only weight-control and exercise interventions, though spouses could also participate.
- Group D—Control group; no programs available.

Planned comparisons among the four study groups included the cost of medical care; number of hospital admissions; number of physician visits; number of and kinds of major disease diagnoses; measurable lifestyle changes (i.e., weight loss, smoking cessation, regular exercise, etc.); number and type of medical problems that occur in those perceived to be more healthy (e.g., nonsmokers vs. smokers; obese vs. ideal weight;

employees under stress vs. those under minimal stress); the effect of dependent participation; effectiveness of regular, supervised exercise; absenteeism due to illness; job turnover; and feelings of well-being and job satisfaction. In all, this project generated nearly 2 million pieces of data, which are currently being analyzed.

In addition to the medical screening, in-depth behavioral modification intervention programs were offered on nutrition; weight loss; smoking cessation; blood pressure control; cholesterol/triglyceride reduction; and preventing back injuries. With the exception of back injury prevention, these programs were conducted on the employees' time, usually immediately after work. All intervention programs were conducted by the professional staffs of the university and Wellness South at fire stations, police precincts, recreation centers, city hall, the fitness center, and other worksite locations.

From the beginning, it was recognized that sometimes several attempts at lifestyle change are required to achieve success, so numerous incentives were provided to encourage active, ongoing participation in the health promotion program. For example, participants received "good health dollars" for attending intervention programs and accomplishing their personal goals. Good health dollars were actually gift certificates printed and provided by a large discount department store. Employees also received T-shirts, gym bags, and certificates of achievement. At the end of the first year, a name was drawn from all employees who participated in intervention programs, and the winner received an expense-paid trip for two to the Caribbean.

Program Results

This 5-year, $3-million effort to evaluate several approaches to medical benefits cost-containment brought together four organizations: the National Institutes of Health, a major teaching university, a private health promotion consulting firm, and the city's employees and their dependents. It was a multiphase approach to medical benefits cost containment. It included a comprehensive, scientific health promotion program and a redesign of the traditional medical plan. During the 5-year project, managed care became available for the first time and was selected by the majority of employees. The overall and per-employee cost savings are well-defined and impressive; however, the value of each of the several cost-containment efforts are more difficult to determine, given that the program findings have not yet been fully analyzed.

No Increase in Medical Benefits Expenses

In 1985, the cost per employee for medical benefits through the city of Birmingham was $2,047, which was about $300 a year above the national average. In 1990, the cost per employee was $2,075, which was about $1,200 below the national average. Over this 5-year period, the city held its per employee medical benefit costs constant while medical benefits expenses for the average employer doubled (Foster & Higgins, Inc., 1992).

Table 9.1 shows that from 1985 to 1990, the number of full-time employees increased from 3,586 to 4,000, while medical expenses increased from $7,342,240 to $8,303,065. Included in these expenses are employer and employee contributions, reserve funds, and administrative fees.

Employee enrollment remained constant at about 76% family and 24% individual. Employee financial contributions increased slightly. During the entire 5-year period, the city paid 100% of individual employee coverage. In 1985, the city paid 86% of family coverage, which decreased to 81% in 1990. This represents an overall increase in employee financial contribution of about 2.9%.

Availability of Managed Care Services

At the beginning of the project, the city started a self-insured, self-administered medical benefits plan. About 6 months later, an HMO became available and was offered as an option to the self-administered indemnity plan. The first year, approximately 63% of the employees selected the HMO over the indemnity plan. Over the next several years, employee preference for the HMO increased to over 90%. Because of this, in 1988, the city ended the indemnity plan and provided medical benefits exclusively through several managed care plans.

Table 9.1
Medical Benefits Expenses Over 5-Year Period (1985–1990)

Fiscal year ending	Medical expenses ($)	$ Increase (or decrease)	% Increase (or decrease)	Full-time positions	Cost per employee ($/yr)
6-30-85	7,342,240	—	—	3,586	2,047
6-30-86	7,633,058	290,818	4.0	3,661	2,084
6-30-87	7,461,646	(171,412)	(2.2)	3,841	1,943
6-30-88	7,886,002	424,356	5.7	3,890	2,027
6-30-89	8,072,113	186,111	2.4	3,932	2,053
6-30-90	8,303,065	231,852	2.9	4,000	2,075

Note. Data from Personnel Department, City of Birmingham, AL.

During the time that both the indemnity plan and HMO were available, the HMO, on average, cost about $18 less per month for a family membership. This financial difference may have been a factor in the selection of managed care over the indemnity plan.

Impact of the All-Employee Medical Screen

The first medical screening, in which nearly all employees participated, revealed that 13% had medical findings serious enough to require referral to a physician. Indicators for physician referral included blood pressure above 170/105 mmHg, cholesterol over 280 mg/dl, HDL-cholesterol under 30 mg/dl, triglycerides over 500 mg/dl, and glucose over 200 mg/dl.

Identifying this group of high-risk employees (many of whom exhibited multiple risk factors as previously described plus obesity, smoking, and heredity) and providing them with proper primary medical management is one of the major reasons for the level of cost containment achieved through this project. Providing proper medical care that will eliminate or minimize risk factors through therapeutic management is an important adjunct to promoting lifestyle change. This is possible only with an all-employee medical screen.

At the all-employee medical screen, employees were asked three confidential questions about their patient-physician relationship: whether they had a regular doctor; whether they would like help in finding a good doctor; and how long it had been since they last visited the doctor. (To assure complete confidentiality, no name or other means of identification was requested.) Analysis of the data indicated that approximately 43% of the employees did not have a regular doctor, but only 17% wanted help in finding a good doctor. The average time since the last doctor visit was 35 months. These data were unexpected and suggested that the health promotion program include a component that teaches employees how to locate and select a primary care physician and how to use the medical benefits plan. Employees were also motivated to have regular preventive-type physical exams. The lack of a copayment for office visits encouraged employees to consult their physicians so that correctable medical problems could be diagnosed and treated before they became catastrophic illnesses.

The personal medical screen data were entered into the computer, and a master list was created that identified each employee, by name, according to risk factors. This confidential list allowed the providers to quickly and accurately identify at-risk employees, who needed individual consultation, and to personally invite them to participate in group intervention programs.

Program Impact

That the city saw no increase in the per-employee cost of medical benefits over a 5-year period is the most important indication of program impact. Another way to gauge program impact is to compare the city's actual cost per employee with the national average per-employee cost. However, when making such comparisons, one must first ask if costs for medical care in Alabama approximate average costs across the country. In 1990, per capita cost for medical care ranged from a high of $3,031 in Massachusetts to a low of $1,689 in South Carolina. In Alabama, the average cost was $2,386, which compares very favorably with the national average of $2,425 and validates the comparison (Families USA Foundation, 1991).

Based on this comparison, total medical benefits expenses were $395,358 above the national average during 1986; $1,119,148 below the national average during 1987; $1,932,358 below the national average during 1988; $3,141,951 below the national average during 1989; and $4,696,935 below the average during 1990. Table 9.2 shows a net savings, for 1985 to 1990, of $10,495,124 compared to the national average. For the 5-year period, actual medical benefits expenses were 21.1% below the national, per-employee average.

Table 9.2
Actual Per-Employee Medical Benefits Expenses
Compared to National Per-Employee Expenses for 1985–1990

Fiscal year ending	City cost/ employee ($)	National average cost/ employee ($)	Forecast* ($)	Actual expenses ($)	$ Increase (or decrease)	% Increase (or decrease)
6-30-85	2,047	1,750				
6-30-86	2,084	1,977	7,237,790	7,633,058	395,268	5.5
6-30-87	1,943	2,234	8,580,794	7,461,646	(1,119,148)	(13.0)
6-30-88	2,027	2,524	9,818,360	7,886,002	(1,932,358)	(19.7)
6-30-89	2,053	2,852	11,214,064	8,072,113	(3,141,951)	(28.0)
6-30-90	2,075	3,250	13,000,000	8,303,065	(4,696,935)	(36.1)
5-yr totals			49,851,008	39,355,884	(10,495,124)	(21.1)

*Forecast based on national average cost per employee, times number of employees.

Note. Data from Personnel Department, City of Birmingham, AL; and from "Health Care Benefits Survey of 2,049 Employees 1991," by A. Foster Higgins & Co., Inc., 1992, Business and Health, **March**.

Employers often ask how long it takes a cost-containment program to become effective. How soon will medical benefit expenses be at or below national average levels? Do reductions in total employee medical expenses level off at some point? When the financial statistics from Table 9.2 are converted to a graphic illustration, there is a clearly defined, nearly stairstep pattern. Figure 9.2 shows that for the city it was several years before per-employee expenses were brought to national average levels, but then, for the next several years, there was a clear geometric progression in cost reductions *below* the national level.

Several factors that may have influenced the economic outcome of this project include

- a medical screen that was a prerequisite for the medical benefits plan,
- identification of those at high risk with aggressive primary care physician referral,
- in-depth intervention programs,
- managed care, and
- plan redesign.

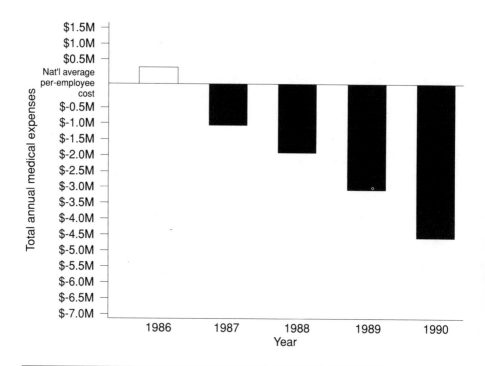

Figure 9.2 Total annual medical expenses, Birmingham compared with national averages. *Note.* Data from Personnel Department, City of Birmingham, AL.

In the final analysis, all of these activities were important, but specific evaluation of the impact of each is not possible. One retrospective way to attempt evaluation of the health promotion program's impact is to recognize that numerous employers in Birmingham from 1985 to 1990 used managed care and redesigned the medical plan along the same lines as the city had. The main difference is that none of the other employers had a health promotion program of the magnitude provided city employees. Conversations with other major employers in the city revealed that none showed a decrease in the cost of medical benefits for the period of 1985 through 1990. In fact, nearly all reported double digit increases during this period.

Program Expenses

This project was not a typical, employer-sponsored health promotion program. It was a controlled experiment, which created systems to collect, store, analyze, and produce large amounts of comparative data. For this reason, approximately $1 million of the total $3-million budget was used to generate protocols, formulate and write computer programs, and input, retrieve, and analyze experimental data. In 1984, there were no computer programs that could handle comparative data of this magnitude. So extensive, costly, and time-consuming computer programming was required.

The remaining $2 million, which amounted to $400,000 annually over 5 years, was used for marketing, promotion, medical screenings, education, and intervention programs. These expenses are not factored into the financial summary in Table 9.2

Unique Aspects of the Birmingham Program

Numerous employers across the country have comprehensive employee health promotion programs. Many are similar to the city of Birmingham program in that they conduct medical screenings and offer intervention programs. Nearly all have redesigned the medical plan, and many have managed medical care. However, they differ in that the city program resulted in no increase in the cost of medical benefits over 5 years, whereas most other employers still experience double-digit annual increases.

With such a dichotomy, the question arises, did the city program contain activities that were unique to the project and, therefore, not a part of other health promotion programs. A retrospective evaluation of the city project suggests that four of its activities are not routinely included in other comprehensive health promotion programs:

1. *Screening of all employees*. This exposes the entire work force to the health promotion program and informs them about personal risk factors.

It is an essential tool, which shows program providers who the multiple-risk employees are so that they can offer individual consultations, follow-up, and intervention.

2. *Aggressive physician referral.* The all-employee medical screening identifies those employees who require immediate physician referral, which in this study was about 13% of all employees tested during the first year. Getting these very high-risk employees under successful medical management is an important adjunct to effective behavioral modification.

3. *Assistance in establishing patient-physician relationships.* Not all employees know how to enter or use the medical benefits plan. Furthermore, this project showed that over 40% of employees did not have an active patient-physician relationship. Education and information programs must help employees understand and become comfortable in establishing an effective patient-physician relationship.

4. *Encouragement of regular physician office visits.* In an effort to reduce utilization costs, many employers have redesigned their medical benefits plans to increase copayments for office visits. But employees who have controllable medical conditions, such as hypertension, diabetes, asthma, high cholesterol, low-HDL, or high triglyceride/low-HDL, should be educated and even encouraged and rewarded for seeing their primary care physicians regularly. Correcting or monitoring medical problems through therapeutic management, in order to prevent catastrophic illnesses or premature death, is an important part of cost-effective health promotion.

These four health promotion activities combined with traditional intervention programs that encourage long-term lifestyle changes offer employers a major opportunity to contain medical benefits costs. Incorporating more traditional efforts, such as plan redesign and managed care, will maximize their cost savings.

The major contributions made to worksite health promotion by the city of Birmingham project were the validation of cost savings, which was illustrated by no increases in medical benefit expenses over the 5 years of the study, and the introduction and successful application of an all-employee medical screening.

Acknowledgments

This study was supported by NIH Grant 5R18HL35105 from the Department of Health and Human Services, National Heart, Lung, and Blood Institute. Special thanks are extended to Mary R. Harvey, Gordon Graham, and Joni Perley for their involvement in this project.

References

Bureau of the Census. (1991, August). *United States census—1990*. Washington, DC: U.S. Government Printing Office.

Castelli, W.P. (1992, May 12). Castelli speaks from the heart. *Fortune*, p. 16.

Data Watch. (1992, July). A snapshot of executive poll results. *Business & Health*, p. 14.

Edington, D. (1992). AFB practitioners forum. *American Journal of Health Promotion*, **6**(6), 403-406.

Families USA Foundation. (1991, July 23). Health cost troubling. *Wall Street Journal*, p. 6.

Foster & Higgins, Inc. (1992, March). Health care benefits survey of 2,049 employers, 1991. *Business & Health*.

Foster & Higgins, Inc. (1983, June). Feasibility study for the city of Birmingham. Birmingham, AL: Author.

Issues & Trends. (1992, June). Executives rating of the top 5 health care concerns. *Business & Health*, p. 18.

Jones, R., Samkoff, J., Wolff, C., & Bowers, T. (1991). Employees health promotion at a university medical center: A pilot project. *American Journal of Health Promotion*, **6**(1), 7-9.

News Briefs. (1991, November). Executives feel lack of control. *Business & Health*, p. 5.

Personnel Department. (1992). Personnel data on file. Birmingham, AL: City of Birmingham.

Chapter 10

A Health Promotion Program for Educators: Hurst-Euless-Bedford Independent School District

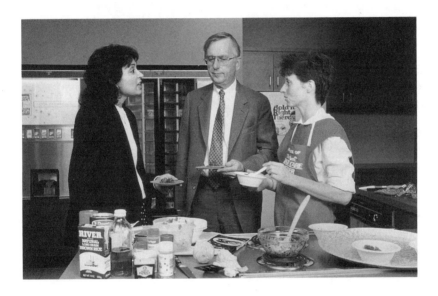

Todd Rogers

Local school districts, collectively, are among the largest employers in the nation; in many localities, schools employ more people than any other business. As is the case for other employers, most school district efforts to stem ever-increasing employee medical care costs are focused on "access control" (cost-sharing, managed care, etc.) rather than "demand reduction" (health promotion programs). Many school district administrators, however, have looked to health promotion programs as a way to contain employee medical care and absenteeism costs (Blair, Tritsch, & Kutsch,

1987; Comprehensive Health Education Resource Center, 1989) and with good reason. With tax revenues declining, school districts generally have experienced minimal budget growth over the past decade while being burdened by rising medical care costs among their employees. Absenteeism also has a direct economic impact on school districts, because costs to hire substitute teachers can be a significant budget item. And the educational model followed by most worksite health promotion programs also tends to fit well with the capabilities of school employees and the physical facilities available to school districts.

Although some studies have documented the cost-containment effects of worksite health promotion programs, criticisms regarding their execution have led some reviewers to caution that the economic argument for offering worksite health promotion is weak and inconsistent (cf. Opatz, Chenoweth, & Kaman, 1991; Warner, 1987; Warner, Wickizer, Wolfe, Schildroth, & Samuelson, 1988). According to Opatz, Chenoweth, and Kaman, there is moderate empirical support for the short-term economic impact of health promotion programs on medical care costs, but the data relating to potential long-term impact on these costs are inconclusive. For absenteeism, the short-term data on the impact of health promotion programs are moderately to strongly supportive, whereas long-term data are inconclusive.

At least one worksite health promotion program for educators has documented improvements in health behavior, fitness, and well-being, as well as reductions in absenteeism (Blair et al., 1984; Blair, Collingwood, Smith, Upton, & Sterling, 1985; Blair et al.,1986). Another has shown that a workplace health promotion program may improve the morale of teachers (Allegrante & Michela, 1990). Few other health promotion programs for educators have been evaluated, and none have demonstrated the impact of the program on medical care costs or presented a cost-benefit analysis of their effects.

The "Heart at Work" Program

Due to rapidly rising costs for health insurance, death benefits, and absenteeism, the administrators of a Texas school district decided to implement and evaluate a pilot worksite health promotion program for employees. With the advice of consultants, district administrators selected the "Heart at Work" (HAW) program, a comprehensive, modular set of guides and materials for worksite health promotion developed and distributed by the American Heart Association (AHA, 1984, 1987; Carpenter, 1988; "Heart at Work," 1985; Leclerc, Gottlieb, & Gaffney, 1986). The HAW program formed the core of the district's health promotion efforts. The focus of this report is on the differential cost-benefit effects of the HAW materials presented as part of a single health risk screening and health education intervention or as part of a comprehensive health promotion program for teachers and staff of the district. The central question was, Is it more cost-beneficial to conduct a relatively simple health screening, counseling, and self-help program than it is to offer a comprehensive health promotion program for school district employees?

The H-E-B Independent School District

The Hurst-Euless-Bedford Independent School District serves a community of approximately 100,000 people in northeast Tarrant County, Texas, midway between Dallas and Fort Worth. During this study, the district consisted of more than 17,000 students enrolled in 17 elementary, 5 junior high, and 2 senior high schools. Of the 1,500 district employees, 1,000 were professional staff members, and more than 50% of the professional staff had advanced degrees. (Note that all demographic, absentee, and insurance usage data were obtained from the district administration; strictest confidentiality procedures were followed, and all participants understood the nature of the project and voluntarily agreed to participate.)

Research Design

Twelve district worksites (11 schools, 1 administrative office building) were randomly assigned from stratified blocks to one of three groups: the high-level (HL) group, which received the greatest amount of training the program offered, consisted of one high school, one junior high school, and four elementary schools with a total workforce of approximately 285 teachers; the low-level (LL) group, which received the least amount of training the program offered, consisted of one high school, one junior high school, and one elementary school with a total workforce of approximately 188 teachers; and the delayed treatment control (DTC) group consisted of the administrative office building, one junior high school, and one elementary school with a total workforce of approximately 145 teachers and staff. Randomization of the worksites ensured that there were no differences among the groups on essential employee characteristics. Due to budgetary constraints, the number of participants was limited by the district administration, so only 305 (49%) of the eligible teachers and staff at these 12 worksites were able to participate in the program. For the present analysis, data on 297 individuals are available (145 HL, 82 LL, and 70 DTC). Missing data are due to individuals leaving the district at midyear ($n = 3$), becoming pregnant ($n = 2$), or not having been employed by the district during the previous (base) year ($n = 3$).

Coordinator Training Program

During the summer before program implementation, one teacher or staff member from each of the HL and LL worksites participated in a comprehensive training program designed to provide them with the basic skills needed to serve as an HAW program coordinator. The HAW program is organized into five modules: high blood pressure; smoking; nutrition; exercise; and signals and actions for survival (heart-attack early warning signs and emergency responses). Each module contains a detailed guide to assist a lay program coordinator in the design and implementation of the most appropriate program for the worksite. Modules are structured so that implementation can be conducted at low, medium, or high levels depending on the assessed needs of the organization. Other HAW guidebooks provide general information on program promotion and evaluation and ways in which local health care providers can support worksite activities (AHA, 1984, 1987).

The volunteer coordinators were provided with more than 40 hours of training before the start of the program and with periodic support throughout the course of the project. Training consisted of didactic and participatory sessions that covered cardiovascular disease epidemiology and prevention, health behavior change and problem solving, and specific intervention approaches for smoking cessation, high blood pressure, exercise, diet, weight control, stress management, and heart-attack early warning signs. Trainees were also taught how to conduct safe and effective group aerobic exercise programs. DTC program coordinators were trained just before the start of the program at their worksites, during the spring semester. All program coordinators received salary supplements from the school district.

Health Screening

In August and September, HL and LL participants went through a detailed, three-stage health and fitness assessment process (Table 10.1). As part of this process, HL and LL participants attended an individual counseling session in which the complete package of HAW and other health education materials was presented. Materials distributed included items from each module of the HAW program. HL participants were given personalized feedback about their health and fitness status and were introduced to the health promotion program that was scheduled to begin immediately at their worksites. LL participants were instructed at the counseling session to follow their individual exercise and behavior change programs until the group program began at their sites in the spring. DTC participants, who served as a control group for the research design, were unaware of their sites' selection into the program until they were invited

Table 10.1
Health and Fitness Assessment

Stage	Assessment method
1	Health history questionnaire
	Blood test & urinalysis
	Body composition analysis
	Resting heart rate & blood pressure
	Pulmonary function test
	Musculoskeletal analysis
	Computerized dietary assessment
	Stool guaiac test
2	Medical review board
3	Health & nutrition consultation
	Distribution of Heart At Work materials

to participate in a health screening and group program during the spring semester.

Health Promotion Program

After the assessment process, the trained coordinators began the HAW program for participants at the three HL worksites. They distributed posters, newsletters, and other printed materials from the AHA and other voluntary health agencies; held brief weekly seminars on health behavior change topics; led 1-hour aerobic exercise classes three times each week; sponsored monthly extended seminars that were conducted by community resource representatives; organized special interest group meetings for walking, weight loss, and other topics; scheduled weigh-ins and blood pressure checks by school nurses; supervised participant self-monitoring and the reward system for wellness activity points and program participation; and coordinated fun runs, fitness festivals, and special meals.

Repeat Assessment

As DTC participants went through their initial health and fitness assessments, HL and LL participants were retested. This repeat assessment included a subset of the initial testing procedures, focusing on measurement of health and fitness variables that had been expected to show changes during the initial intervention period (e.g., body composition, blood pressure, fitness levels, dietary habits, and self-reported health behaviors).

After their health and fitness assessment, DTC participants joined a high-level HAW program, which was conducted at their worksites. This program was identical to that made available to HL participants. LL participants also had a high-level HAW program conducted at their worksites during this second phase of intervention. HL participants were then phased into a maintenance program with fewer activities available.

Calculating Program Costs and Benefits

Program costs included only those costs associated directly with program administration (i.e., health and fitness assessments, coordinators' salaries and training, program activities and materials, and central administrative costs). Indirect costs were not included, because office space, furniture, utilities, and the like were not additional costs required for running the program, and the classrooms used would have stood empty had the program not been conducted. Because the district was interested in the *operational* costs and benefits of the program, fees for evaluation research and consulting also were not included. Participant contributions to the program were deducted from the direct costs. Contributions from each program participant during the entire year were $143, $113, and $90 for HL, LL, and DTC participants, respectively.

Program benefits were measured by reviewing absenteeism data obtained from the school district and medical care claims data maintained by the district's third-party insurance administrator. Absences due to professional leave or jury duty were excluded from analysis. Costs for absences were calculated by multiplying the days absent by the day rate for substitute teachers, which was $42.00 during the intervention school year. Net medical care claims data were analyzed after adjustment for deductibles and copayments. Data were collected for the program year as well as for the base year before the program, which served as the reference period. Data were also analyzed for the experimental period (September through March of the school year) as well as for the full program year (September through August). All financial data were reported in nondiscounted dollars constant to the base year.

Program Results

Participants at the three participation levels did not differ on basic demographic factors, such as average age (40.7 years, 40.0 years, and 42.0 years), or the proportion of women participants (78%, 73%, and 88%) for HL,

LL, and DTC groups, respectively. Figure 10.1 shows the average dollar amounts of medical insurance claims for each group during the base and program years. Figure 10.2 shows the average number of work absences each year. All subsequent analyses of program-year data are reported using insurance claims and work absence data that have been adjusted for the base-year experience of participants.

Group Differences

Figure 10.3 shows that for HL and LL participants, the average *adjusted* changes in insurance claims during the program year relative to the base year were significantly less than zero ($p < .05$). (Note that the figures shown in Table 10.4 are *not* statistically adjusted.) That is, participants in the HL and LL groups showed a statistically significant drop in medical insurance claims relative to the base year (reductions of $386 and $259, respectively). DTC participants, whose data were retrospectively evaluated after their entry into the program, showed a statistically nonsignificant *increase* of $239 in insurance claims relative to the base year. These increases followed the historical trend of increasing health insurance costs among district employees.

Planned contrast results for the insurance claims data are reported in Table 10.2. The average adjusted changes in medical insurance claims

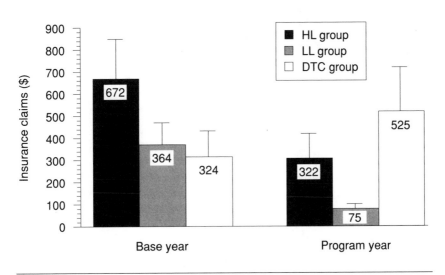

Figure 10.1   Average annual insurance claims by experimental group; mean ± standard error.

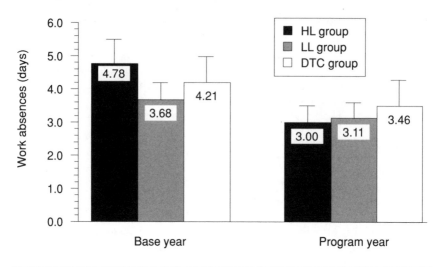

Figure 10.2 Average annual work absences by experimental group; mean ± standard error.

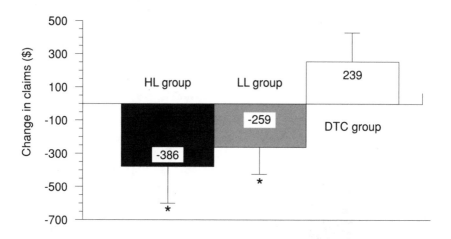

Figure 10.3 Adjusted change in insurance claims from base to program year by experimental group; mean ± standard error. * = significant reduction from base year (p < .05).

(relative to the base year) were significantly different between the HL and DTC groups and between the HL and LL groups combined and the DTC group. (Note that analyses using log transformations of these positively skewed data revealed identical within- and between-group findings. Nonparametric analyses of differences in median changes also were consistent with the parametric findings.)

Table 10.2
Between-Group Planned Contrasts

Planned contrast	Change in adjusted insurance	Change in adjusted absence
High-level vs. low-level	NS	NS
High-level & low-level vs. delayed treatment control	$p < .03$	NS
High-level vs. delayed treatment control	$p < .04$	NS
Low-level vs. delayed treatment control	NS	NS

Note. Data analyzed are changes for entire program year relative to the entire base year, adjusted for prior year experience; planned contrasts are those that were established a priori to have research relevance.

Figure 10.4 presents the adjusted changes in work absences for each group during the program year relative to the base year. Only HL participants showed a statistically significant decline in average absences during this period.

Table 10.2 also presents the planned contrast results for the work absence data. There were no significant between-group differences for adjusted absence changes.

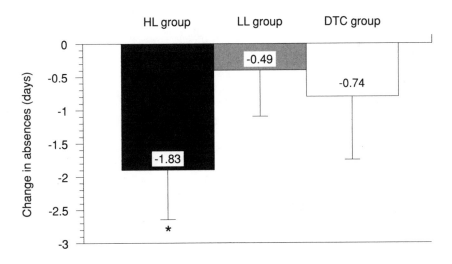

Figure 10.4 Change in adjusted work absences from base to program year by experimental group; mean ± standard error. * = signifcant reduction from base year ($p < .05$).

Analyzing Program Benefits and Costs

Analysis of program costs and benefits were reported in two ways: (a) changes during the 7-month experimental period (September through March) in the program year relative to the same 7-month period during the base year, and (b) changes for the entire program year (September through August) for medical insurance data, and for the entire school year (September through May) for absenteeism data, also relative to the same periods during the base year.

Table 10.3 reports the average economic costs and benefits during the experimental period for the three groups; per-participant analyses are shown in the upper portion of the table, whereas total program costs and benefits are shown in the bottom portion. After deducting the average

Table 10.3
Economic Costs and Benefits for Experimental Period
(in Constant Base-Year Dollars)

Component	High-level group (n = 145)	Low-level group (n = 82)	Control group (n = 70)
Costs per participant			
Direct costs	306.10	239.05	N/A
(Less contributions)	(78.00)	(48.00)	N/A
Net costs	228.10	191.05	0.00
Benefits per participant*			
Medical insurance savings	253.42	160.92	(6.62)
Work absence savings	84.58	28.68	51.87
Total benefits	338.00	189.60	45.25
Benefit:cost ratio	1.48	0.99	N/A
All participant costs			
Direct costs	44,384.50	19,602.10	N/A
(Less contributions)	(11,310.00)	(3,936.00)	N/A
Net costs	33,074.50	15,666.10	0.00
All participant benefits*			
Medical insurance savings	36,745.38	13,195.55	(542.64)
Work absence savings	12,264.04	2,351.91	4,253.00
Total benefits	49,009.42	15,547.45	3,710.35
Total savings (loss)	15,934.92	(118.65)	3,710.35

*Unadjusted cost reductions or increases from base year, same period.

contribution to the program by participants, the average net cost to the district was $228.10 for each participant in the HL group and $191.05 for each member of the LL group. There was no cost for DTC participants during the experimental period.

Average unadjusted benefits for each group during the experimental period are included in Table 10.3. The average HL participant had $338 in medical insurance and work absence reductions relative to the base year, while the average LL participant had about $190 in benefits. The average DTC participant had some savings due to reduced absence levels from the base year which offset increases in medical insurance costs. The benefit-to-cost ratios reported for the HL and LL groups show a net savings only for HL participants. For each dollar directly invested in the HL program, the district got $1.48 in return during the experimental period. The LL program almost broke even during the experimental period.

The bottom portion of Table 10.3 shows all-participant results for the experimental period: The HL group returned to the district nearly $16,000 on a $33,000 net investment after participant contributions; the LL group lost the district about $120 on a $15,666 net investment; and the decline in work absences shown by the DTC group saved the district more than $3,700 without any investment during the experimental period.

Table 10.4 reports the economic costs and benefits for each group for the program. Direct costs were calculated as discussed previously except that posttesting charges for HL and LL participants were included in the direct cost figures. Unadjusted benefits were similarly calculated using the entire base year as the reference. The average HL participant had about $425 in medical insurance and work absence reductions relative to the base year, while the average LL participant had about $313 reduction in benefits. The average DTC participant cost the district about $169 more than during the base year due to increases in medical insurance costs. The benefit-to-cost ratios reported for the HL and LL groups show a net savings for these participants. For each dollar directly invested in the HL program, the district saved $1.37 over the entire year. For each dollar directly invested in the LL program, the district received only $1.02 in return over the entire program year.

The bottom portion of Table 10.4 shows all-participant results for the entire year: The HL group returned more than $16,000 to the district on a $45,000 investment; the LL group yielded about $500 on a $25,000 investment; and the DTC group lost the district more than $28,000 on a $15,000 investment. The DTC group loss was due to the more than $16,000 increase in medical insurance claims during the program year relative to the base year.

Table 10.4
Economic Costs and Benefits for Program Year
(in Constant Base-Year Dollars)

Component	High-level group (n = 145)	Low-level group (n = 82)	Control group (n = 70)
Costs per participant			
Direct costs	452.10	419.20	271.34
(Less contributions)	(143.00)	(113.00)	(90.00)
Net costs	309.10	306.20	181.34
Benefits per participant*			
Medical insurance savings	350.11	288.75	(200.94)
Work absence savings	74.59	23.82	31.80
Total benefits	424.70	312.57	(169.14)
Benefit:cost ratio	1.37	1.02	N/A
All participant costs			
Direct costs	65,554.50	34,374.40	22,249.88
(Less contributions)	(20,735.00)	(9,266.00)	(7,380.00)
Net costs	44,819.50	25,108.40	14,869.88
All participant benefits*			
Medical insurance savings	50,766.24	23,677.59	(16,477.13)
Work absence savings	10,815.23	1,953.09	2,607.45
Total benefits	61,581.47	25,630.68	(13,869.68)
Total savings (loss)	16,761.97	522.28	(28,739.56)

*Unadjusted cost reductions or increases from base year.

What Do the Results Mean?

Opatz et al. (1991) argue that studies of the potential economic impact of health promotion need to address five issues:

1. Generalizability (i.e., conduct studies in businesses other than manufacturing and insurance)
2. Employee population (i.e., focus on individuals other than male, white-collar workers)
3. Worksite size (i.e., look at smaller settings)
4. Cost-effectiveness (i.e., hold off on cost-benefit studies until better methodology for obtaining long-term cost and benefit estimates can be developed)

5. Research design (i.e., use designs that minimize threats to the internal validity of the study)

The present study directly addressed most of these issues: It employed a randomized design with a female-dominated workforce in a relatively small worksite that was not in the manufacturing or insurance sectors.

This study's major limitation is that only short-term costs and benefits were monitored. This is a significant limitation because it is well known that an individual's medical care costs can vary greatly from year to year. The more years in the study, the more stable the cost estimates (Lynch, Teitelbaum, & Main, 1991). And though the sites were randomly assigned to experimental conditions, the individuals working at the sites were allowed to volunteer their participation in the program (the district did impose a limit on the number of participants). Thus, self-selection bias could have influenced these results, assuming that there were differential medical care utilization and absenteeism rates among the volunteers in the three groups. (Note, however, that the retrospective analysis of the DTC group data, with the finding of significant increases in medical care insurance claims consistent with the general experience of the district, argues against a self-selection bias. Presumably, the DTC volunteer participants had the same self-selection predispositions that the HL and LL participants had; yet, the DTC group showed a very unfavorable change in medical care insurance utilization.)

These few concerns notwithstanding, the results of the present analysis suggest the following conclusions: (a) Though a single, health and fitness assessment and counseling procedure, which used HAW materials, yielded significant reductions in medical insurance claims relative to the preceding year, the low-level program did not yield a favorable benefit-to-cost ratio; (b) a full-scale health promotion effort, which used an intensive health and fitness assessment and the HAW program, showed significant within-group reductions in work absences, significantly greater reductions in medical care insurance claims costs compared to a control group, substantial bottom-line savings, and a favorable, short-term benefit-to-cost ratio; and (c) program implementation was successfully accomplished by nonprofessional coordinators who were provided with a training and support program.

The limitations of this study temper any enthusiasm for endorsing full-scale health promotion programs for educators (whether Heart at Work or any other) as a means of slowing rising medical insurance and work absence costs. Future research must answer these and other questions: What are the cost-benefit results of a comprehensive program offered without an extensive health and fitness assessment? Would a less intensive (and therefore, less expensive) health and fitness assessment have been equally effective? Would the program have been as effective without the extensive training and support of the coordinators? And what are the long-term cost-benefit effects of the Heart at Work program or, for that matter, *any* comprehensive worksite health promotion program?

Acknowledgments

This project was completed while the author was with Health Management Consultants, Inc. and the Las Colinas Preventive Medicine Clinic. The study would not have been possible without the dedicated efforts of Jo Ann Cole, Michael Dehn, Dr. Richard Johnston, Janine Maupin, and other members of the clinic staff. Additional support for data analyses and manuscript preparation were provided by the Cooper Institute for Aerobics Research and the Henry J. Kaiser Family Foundation. Finally, many thanks to Pamela Erwin and Troy Green of the Hurst-Euless-Bedford Independent School District, Howard Shiflett of the American Heart Association, and Dr. Steven Blair of the Cooper Institute for Aerobics Research. Preliminary findings were presented in *Heart at Work Technical Report: Extended Field Studies* (American Heart Association, 1987). Address all correspondence to Todd Rogers, PhD, Director, Health Promotion Resource Center, Stanford Center for Research in Disease Prevention, Stanford University School of Medicine, 1000 Welch Road, Palo Alto, CA 94304-1885.

References

Allegrante, J.P., & Michela, J.L. (1990). Impact of a school-based workplace health promotion program on morale of inner-city teachers. *Journal of School Health*, **60**, 25-28.

American Heart Association. (1984). *Heart at Work technical report.* Dallas: Author.

American Heart Association. (1987). *Heart at Work technical report: Extended field studies.* Dallas: Author.

Blair, S.N., Collingwood, T.R., Reynolds, R., Smith, M., Hagan, D.R., & Sterling, C.L. (1984). Health promotion for educators: Impact on health behaviors, satisfaction, and general well-being. *American Journal of Public Health*, **74**, 147-149.

Blair, S.N., Collingwood, T.R., Smith, M., Upton, J., & Sterling, C.L. (1985). Review of a health promotion program for school employees. *Special Services in the Schools*, **1**, 89-97.

Blair, S.N., Smith, M., Collingwood, T.R., Reynolds, R., Prentice, M.C., & Sterling, C.L. (1986). Health promotion for educators: Impact on absenteeism. *Preventive Medicine*, **15**, 166-175.

Blair, S.N., Tritsch, L., & Kutsch, S. (1987). Worksite health promotion for school faculty and staff. *Journal of School Health, 57,* 469-473.

Carpenter, R.A. (1988). Heart at Work: The evaluation of a low-cost worksite health promotion program. *American Association of Occupational Health Nursing Journal, 36,* 276-281.

Comprehensive Health Education Resource Center. (1989). *School site health promotion: An ideabook.* Sacramento: California Department of Health Services.

"Heart at Work" campaign encourages healthier living. (1985). *Journal of the American Medical Association, 254,* 1422-1423.

Leclerc, K.M., Gottlieb, N.H., & Gaffney, C. (1986). Application of the Heart at Work module to a worksite health promotion program. *American Association of Occupational Health Nursing Journal, 34,* 370-376.

Lynch, W.D., Teitelbaum, H.S., & Main, D.S. (1991). The inadequacy of using means to compare medical costs of smokers and nonsmokers. *American Journal of Health Promotion, 6,* 123-128.

Opatz, J., Chenoweth, D., & Kaman, R. (1991, August). *Economic impact of worksite health promotion.* (Available from: Association for Worksite Health Promotion, 310 North Alabama Street, Suite A100, Indianapolis, IN 46204.)

Warner, K.E. (1987). Selling health promotion to corporate America: Uses and abuses of the economic argument. *Health Education Quarterly, 14,* 39-55.

Warner, K.E., Wickizer, T.M., Wolfe, R.A., Schildroth, J.E., & Samuelson, M.H. (1988). Economic implications of workplace health promotion programs: Review of the literature. *Journal of Occupational Medicine, 30,* 106-112.

Chapter 11

The LIVE FOR LIFE® Program of Johnson & Johnson: Direct and Indirect Economic Benefits

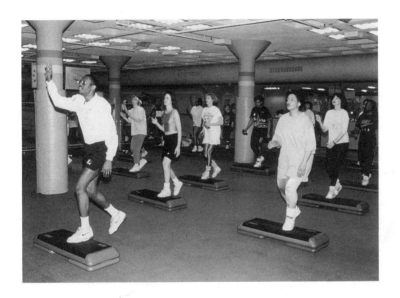

Jonathan E. Fielding

During the late 1970s consensus developed among biomedical, academic, and government communities that individual health habits were major contributors to many of the common causes of premature death and disability. Smoking, poor diet, lack of regular exercise, and elevated cholesterol were linked to cardiovascular disease, cerebrovascular disease, and cancer, the cause of about two thirds of all deaths in the United States (National Center for Health Statistics, 1992). Results from clinical risk reduction studies and from such community interventions as the Stanford Three Community Study, the North Karelia Project, Multiple Risk Factor

Intervention Trial (MRFIT), and others suggested that the lifestyles of large numbers of people could be altered (Kornitzer, DeBacker, Dramaix, & Kittel, 1983; Maccoby, Farquhar, Wood, & Alexander, 1977; MRFIT Research Group, 1982; Salonen, Puska, Kottke, & Tuomilehto, 1981). During the same period, the notion that health was a positive attribute that could contribute to personal productivity gained credence. Meanwhile both the public and private sectors were under increasing pressure to develop effective strategies to moderate the rate of increase of health care costs and other consequences of ill health, such as absenteeism and disability.

LIVE FOR LIFE: Origin, Rationale, and Structure

By the late 1970s Johnson & Johnson, like most major private and public employers, offered a comprehensive health benefit plan and paid the vast majority of plan costs for employees and dependents through a largely self-insured health benefit plan. Johnson & Johnson's health benefit costs were rising more rapidly than most other costs borne by the corporation and were cause for concern. In 1980, illness costs alone represented 2.3% of net sales, a 35% increase over 1977 levels. Even at a conservatively projected 13% annual increase, illness-care costs were projected to double between 1981 and 1989 (Benefits Department, Johnson & Johnson, personal communication, 1980).

Opportunities to improve the health and well-being of its employees were of particular interest to Johnson & Johnson in light of its position as the largest and most diversified manufacturer of health care products worldwide. As the scientific evidence linking lifestyle and health and the benefits of reducing health risks accumulated, Johnson & Johnson decided to test the feasibility of improving health through employer-sponsored lifestyle change programs. Johnson & Johnson's decision was influenced by the credo that guides the company, which states in part that management is "responsible to our employees." James E. Burke, then chairman and chief executive officer of Johnson & Johnson, decided to provide Johnson & Johnson employees with all the resources necessary to become the healthiest employee population of any corporation in the world. Mr. Burke indicated that it would be illogical for a health care company not to have healthy employees.

The LIVE FOR LIFE program was conceived in response to Mr. Burke's challenge. As originally implemented, the Johnson & Johnson program was coordinated by a volunteer task force of employees. Later, this evolved into a structure with an account manager for each participating operating company. All employees were encouraged to take a nurse-administered health profile, which included behavioral, attitudinal, and biometric measures (blood pressure, blood lipids, body fat, height and weight, and submaximal exercise testing using bicycle ergometry; see Figure 11.1). The health profile, which required 1 hour to complete, was offered on company time.

Employees were then invited to participate in a 3-hour lifestyle seminar to introduce them to all aspects of the LIVE FOR LIFE program and afford them the opportunity to ask questions about the program or the relationship of lifestyle to health problems. The core of lifestyle improvement activities at the outset included behaviorally oriented programs dealing with nutrition, exercise, weight control, smoking cessation, stress management, blood pressure control, and other risk factors usually identified as important by the health coordinator at each site.

As part of the health seminar, the importance of regular exercise was emphasized. In a limited number of work locations, employees were given an opportunity to exercise on their own time at company-provided fitness facilities. Incentives, including clothing and sports equipment, were offered to reward participation in the activities. Employees were also encouraged to become involved in all the various aspects of the program. Promotion of the entire program and specific events were aimed at maximizing employee participation.

The program was conceived as influencing all Johnson & Johnson employees, regardless of whether they formally participated in specific LIVE FOR LIFE activities (see Figure 11.2). It was assumed that due to different personal learning styles and preferences, some employees would prefer to undertake risk-reducing activities, such as regular exercise or smoking cessation, outside of a formal program. Therefore the promotional efforts were designed to motivate individuals to change with or without the assistance of formal programs. LIVE FOR LIFE incorporated efforts to shift the employees' entire environment toward health, structurally and socially.

Johnson & Johnson is a decentralized company, and the decision to adopt the program was at the discretion of each operating company. Initially, only a few companies indicated a strong interest in this nascent concept. During the first 3 to 4 years of its existence, LIVE FOR LIFE was a demonstration and evaluation project with a subsegment of interested Johnson & Johnson operating companies as intervention sites; other sites served as controls until data collection for the initial series of studies had been completed.

The mission and programming of LIVE FOR LIFE has undergone a significant evolution since its inception. Through careful formative and summative assessment of the program, a number of opportunities for program improvement and refinement were identified. By 1984 the mission had been refined to providing the direction and resources to Johnson & Johnson employees, families, and communities that would result in healthier lifestyles and help contain illness care costs.

Health practices	My score	Excellent	Good	Needs self-improvement	Requires change	Requires immediate action
Cigarette smoking		*Nonsmoker 1 year or more	Nonsmoker < 1 year	1-3 cigarettes per day	4-9 cigarettes per day	10+ cigarettes per day
Pipe smoking		*Current nonsmoker	N/A	1 bowl/day	2-3 bowls per day	4+ bowls per day
Cigar smoking		*Current nonsmoker	N/A	1 cigar/day	2-3 cigars per day	4+ cigars per day
Smokeless tobacco		*No regular use	N/A	N/A	Regular use	N/A
Eating practices						
Fat/cholesterol	97	*92 or more	88-91	81-87	61-80	60 or less
Salt	98	100	*94-99	86-93	77-85	76 or less
Fiber	74	*48 or more	34-37	20-33	12-19	11 or less
Sugar	94	*94 or more	88-93	66-87	53-65	52 or less
High-vitamin vegetables	17	28 or more	*16-27	9-15	5-8	4 or less
Dental practices		*Checkup, brush, and floss	N/A	Checkup and brush, no floss	Brush, no floss or checkup	No checkup, brush, or floss
Self-care	52	90 or more	70-89	*45-69	20-44	19 or less
Home safety	59	80 or more	60-79	*40-59	20-39	19 or less
Motor vehicle safety					****	
General well-being		****				

Health practices	My score	Excellent	Good	Needs self-improvement	Requires change	Requires immediate action
Level of stress				****		
Managing stress						
Coping style		****				
Relationships/support			****			
Healthy heart behavior			****			
Aerobic exercises or physical activity		4 or more	3	*2	1 or less	Not at all
(Calories per week)	1,400	3,000+	2,000-2,999	*1,000-1,999	500-999	499 or less
Health measures						
Systolic blood pressure	100	*120 or less	121-130	131-140	141-150	151 or more
Diastolic blood pressure	62	*80 or less	81-85	86-90	91-95	96 or more
Percent above ideal body weight	6%	5% or less	*6-10%	11-20%	21-29%	30% or more
Percent body fat	23%	*25% or less	26-28%	29-36%	37-39%	40% or more
Fitness aerobic capacity	46	*42 or more	31-41	24-30	17-23	16 or less

I.D. Number:
Health score:
Health potential: 1,000

*Indicates your score.

Figure 11.1 Sample LIVE FOR LIFE Health Profile. *Note.* Data from Johnson & Johnson Health Management, Inc.

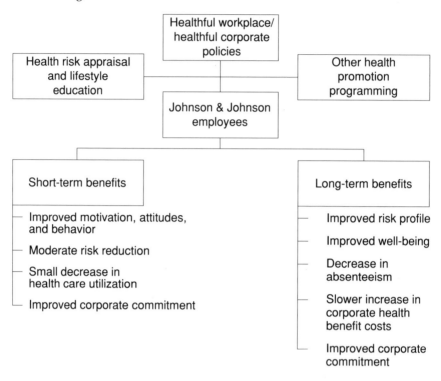

Figure 11.2   LIVE FOR LIFE conceptualization of program effects.

The program has grown to reach over 28,000 domestic employees of Johnson & Johnson. Periodic employee surveys consistently identify LIVE FOR LIFE as one of the most highly prized benefits, and the programming is viewed as very positive (A. Herrmann, personal communication, May 1992). Because of this positive perception, it was decided to make LIVE FOR LIFE the banner for a wide variety of employee benefits and medical programs. LIVE FOR LIFE is thus an umbrella title, not only for the wellness program, but also for occupational health, the medical portion of the employee benefit plan, the employee assistance program, and the safety program. The broadened concept of LIVE FOR LIFE facilitates benefits integration and communication about various benefits to employees and their families.

Evaluation Design and Methodologies

With the help of behavioral scientists, epidemiologists, and health promotion experts, a plan for the development and testing of a comprehensive health promotion program was crafted. The evaluation plan was designed to assess program impact on entire worksites, and an explicit program objective was to influence all employees, despite variation in the extent of individual participation in formal program activities. Ideally, a worksite health promotion program evaluation considers effects on health knowledge, health risk factors, health status, mortality, economic aspects, and measures of productivity (Breslow, Fielding, Herrmann, & Wilbur, 1990). The time allotted for observation of possible impact from the interventions, the number of persons in the intervention and comparison groups, and the circumstances of initiating the program permitted assessment of all components except mortality. Methodological barriers to direct measurement of most aspects of productivity in work settings left only direct measurement of absenteesim and company and job-related attitudes as productivity measures. Some of the data pertain to different cohorts of employees, in particular those concerning health-related variables and those that are measures of economic impact.

Effects on Health

A quasi-experimental design was maintained for 2 years among two sets of Johnson & Johnson manufacturing plants with comparable demographics and job-class distributions and located within a 50-mile radius of each other in central New Jersey and northern Pennsylvania. Plants that were part of four Johnson & Johnson companies introduced the entire LIVE FOR LIFE program to 2,600 employees, whereas those of three companies offered only the health screening component to 1,700 employees. It should be noted that the health-screening-only component included administration of the 1-hour health profile by a specially trained nurse-consultant plus a group seminar; thus the control condition was a significant intervention. Therefore, any findings of intergroup differences where greater change was observed in the intervention groups should be considered conservative.

About 75% of all employees at both sets of plants completed the voluntary health screening at baseline. An additional random sample of employees who had not volunteered but were also surveyed had a 65% response rate (Health Profile Non-Respondents, 1981). Respondents and nonrespondents had approximately equivalent health indicators and lifestyle indicators, except that somewhat more nonrespondents reported smoking cigarettes or exercising regularly. Health profile participants appeared to reflect the demographic characteristics, health status, type of work, and lifestyle characteristics of the entire work force (Settergren, Wilbur, Hartwell, & Rassweiler, 1983).

The primary analyses contrasted the experiences of the intervention and health-screening-only companies. These two populations had similar demographic and health-related characteristics (Wilbur, Hartwell, & Piserchia, 1985). Approximately 95% of both groups provided information at baseline and again at 2 years.

Preliminary findings after the first 12 months (see Table 11.1) indicated that, compared to the control group, the LIVE FOR LIFE group showed improvement in weight, exercise, blood pressure, percent body weight above ideal, cigarette smoking, self-reported sick days, and other characteristics (Wilbur & Garner, 1984).

Table 11.1
Effects of LIVE FOR LIFE Program on Employee Health

| Survey | Measure | Percentage change, baseline-Year 1 | | |
		Intervention	Control	p-value
Year-1 retest	Aerobic calories/kg/wk	+43	+6	0.001
	% above ideal weight	−1	+6	0.001
	% current smokers	−15	−4	0.050
	General well-being	+5	+2	0.001
	% blood pressure ≥ 140/90	−32	−9	NR
	Self-reported sick days	−9	+14	0.050
	Satisfaction with working conditions	+3	−7	0.001

NR = not reported.

Note. From "Marketing Health to Employees, the Johnson & Johnson LIVE FOR LIFE Program" by C.S. Wilber and D. Garner. In *Marketing Health Behavior* by L.W. Frederiksen, L.J. Solomon, and K.A. Breheney, 1984, New York: Plenum Publishing Corporation. Reprinted by permission.

Physical Fitness.   More extensive analysis, which utilized Year 2 data, demonstrated strong differences in change scores for cigarette smoking (Shipley, Orleans, Wilbur, Piserchia, & McFadden, 1988) and exercise and physical fitness (Blair, Piserchia, Wilbur, & Crowder, 1986). In the LIVE FOR LIFE group, approximately 20% of the women and 30% of the men reported achieving a regimen of regular physical exercise, defined as walking or jogging at least 10 miles a week or an equivalent energy expenditure in other vigorous activities or sports (see Table 11.2). Seven percent of women and 19% of men in the control group, who had reported no regular, vigorous physical activity at baseline, achieved the defined fitness threshold. Submaximal bicycle ergometry provided an indirect measure of aerobic capacity at the end of the second year. After 2 years,

Table 11.2
Effects of LIVE FOR LIFE Program on Physical Fitness and Exercise

Measure	Percentage change, baseline-Year 2		
	Intervention	Control	p-value
Daily energy expenditure in vigorous activity	+104.0	+33.0	<0.0001
$\dot{V}O_2$max	+10.5	+4.7	<0.0001

Note. From "A Public Health Intervention Model for Worksite Health Promotion: Impact on Exercise and Physical Fitness in a Health Promotion Plan After 24 Months" by S.N. Blair, P.V. Piserchia, C.S. Wilbur, and J.H. Crowder, 1986, *Journal of the American Medical Association*, **255**, pp. 921-926. Copyright 1986, American Medical Association. Reprinted by permission.

least-squares means for $\dot{V}O_2$max, after adjustment for sex, age, and baseline score, were 38.7 (ml $\times$ kg^{-1} $\times$ min^{-1}) and 36.7 for employees who underwent only the health screening ($p < 0.0001$; Blair et al., 1986). Also the intervention group increased their $\dot{V}O_2$max to 10.5% above baseline versus 4.7% for the control group (Blair et al., 1986). Surveys of the non-respondent group indicated that attrition bias did not account for the intergroup differences.

It is particularly significant that the 10.5% increase in $\dot{V}O_2$max was the average for the entire population of the LIVE FOR LIFE worksites, not just those who volunteered to participate. Also the observed LIVE FOR LIFE site increase approached 50% of the maximum conditioning response seen in laboratory-based programs intended to increase exercise. Changes in self-reported exercise habits and directly ascertainable fitness measures of endurance were distributed throughout the working population at the LIVE FOR LIFE sites. All age groups, whites and nonwhites, all socioeconomic groups, and both married and single groups exhibited such changes (Blair et al., 1986).

Smoking Cessation.   All employees at LIVE FOR LIFE sites identified at baseline were offered a 13-session professionally led smoking cessation program (4 sessions to help smokers prepare for quitting, 5 for quitting, and 4 for maintenance; Shipley et al., 1988). At the control sites, employees were counseled during the health screenings about the importance of quitting but were not offered the formal smoking cessation program.

Baseline level of smoking at LIVE FOR LIFE companies was 27.2%, lower than at the health-screenings-only companies (34.5%), with the primary difference in the never-smoked category (see Table 11.3). However, smokers at both sets of companies were similar in demographic and other health risk characteristics at baseline, except the health-screening-only population was at somewhat higher risk for coronary heart disease.

At LIVE FOR LIFE companies, 22.6% of all smokers quit during the 2-year program. The period of abstinence averaged 14.8 months. In the control group, 17.4% quit and abstinence averaged 12.3 months ($p = 0.12$). In both groups, cessation rates were greater than that of the estimated secular trend, 4% to 5% a year. Thiocyanate validation of self-reported quitting was not complete, but the data available supported the accuracy of the self-reports.

Of all employees at high risk for coronary heart disease, 32% at LIVE FOR LIFE companies quit smoking versus 12.9% at the control sites. Participation in at least one session of the smoking cessation clinic was associated with a 31.6% quit rate at follow-up 2 years later. By contrast, 20.2% of the smoking employees exposed to LIVE FOR LIFE but who did not attend the clinic quit smoking on their own. The quit rate in the comparison group at the control sites was 17.4%.

Table 11.3
Effects of LIVE FOR LIFE Program on Smoking

Measure	Percentage change, baseline—2 years		p-value
	Intervention	Control	
Percentage quit smoking by Year 2	−22.6	−17.4	0.120
Percentage quit smoking by Year 2, high risk for CHD	−32.0	−12.9	<0.010

Note. From "Effect of the Johnson & Johnson LIVE FOR LIFE Program on Employee Smoking" by R.H. Shipley, C.T. Orleans, C.S. Wilbur, P.V. Piserchia, and D.W. McFadden, 1988, Preventive Medicine, 17. Reprinted by permission.

Seat Belt Use.   Seat belt use was recommended to LIVE FOR LIFE program employees through a printed statement on the health screening evaluation form. However, seat belt use was not a primary focus of LIVE FOR LIFE in its early stages, and there was no broad-scale evaluation of changes in seat belt use. However, due to its impact on death and serious injury among Johnson & Johnson employees (and at the suggestion of a Rutgers University faculty member), seat belt use was tested by a low-intensity intervention at one company facility. A 1-week intervention took place at a facility that had its own parking area (Weinstein, Grubb, & Vautier, 1986). During the week, drivers who used the targeted parking facility received memorandums encouraging seat belt use and announcing that dashboard reminder stickers would be provided and that a small gift (a key chain or Frisbee) would be given to drivers who said they used the stickers in their vehicles. In that facility, messages encouraging seat belt use were displayed on cafeteria tables and "Buckle Up" signs were placed on the parking decks.

A nearby parking facility used by employees of one division of the participating Johnson & Johnson company and other predominantly white-collar workers served as a control. Observations at the two parking entrances to the intervention parking lots revealed more frequent use of seat belts by drivers during the 6 weeks after the intervention than preintervention. At a 6-month follow-up the proportion of drivers using their seat belts at this parking lot had further increased to 61% above baseline (i.e., to 50% use) at one entrance and to 33% above baseline (i.e., to 40% use) at the other (see Table 11.4). Seat belt use rates at the control facility remained very close to the preintervention rate of 18.6%.

Table 11.4
Effects of LIVE FOR LIFE Program on Seat Belt Use

	Percentage belt use		p-value (as compared to control group)
	Baseline	6 months	
Control group*	18.6	21.7	NA
North survey site	31.1	50.0	<0.001
South survey site	30.2	40.3	<0.010

NA = Not Applicable.

*Control group included non-J&J employees.

Note. From "Increasing Automobile Seat Belt Use: An Intervention Emphasizing Risk Susceptibility" by N.D. Weinstein, P.D. Grubb, and J.S. Vautier, 1986, *Journal of Applied Psychology*, **71**, pp. 285-290. Copyright 1986 by the American Psychological Association. Reprinted by permission.

Direct Economic Effects

Part of Johnson & Johnson's substantial financial commitment to LIVE FOR LIFE included an analysis of the program's direct economic effects. This involved comparison of the changes in absenteeism and corporate paid health benefit costs between the intervention and control groups.

Changes in Absenteeism Rates.   Absenteeism data from the four LIVE FOR LIFE sites that initiated programs in late 1979 or 1980, which were fully operational throughout 1981, were compared with data from five nearby Johnson & Johnson companies that had no LIVE FOR LIFE program through the end of 1981. Absenteeism data were examined for 3 years, 1979 through 1981 (Jones, Bly, & Richardson, 1990). After 1981 the reliability of data on absenteeism declined, due to a change in federal regulations that exempted wages paid for sick leave from taxation by Social Security.

Data were obtained at all study and control sites on all employees who responded to health and lifestyle questionnaires at baseline and in Year 2 of the program and who had been employed throughout that period. There were 1,406 persons in the LIVE FOR LIFE group and 487 in the control group. Although limitations on employees included introduced potential bias, this design permitted consideration of self-reported sick days, smoking status, and other lifestyle variables in what were considered important extensions of the primary analyses. No data were available on extent of participation of employees at LIVE FOR LIFE companies.

Preliminary examination of the data revealed differences between the two study groups in age, gender, job classification (wage-earning or salaried) distributions, and baseline (1979) absenteeism. Intergroup differences were controlled for by employing separate regressions for wage-earning and salaried personnel and by using analyses of covariance.

After controlling for age, gender, and baseline differences, the adjusted mean absentee hours for both groups of wage-earning employees were very similar in 1980. In 1981, however, the LIVE FOR LIFE group displayed a significantly lower mean level of excludable sick hours ($p < .01$; see Table 11.5). Adjusted mean hours increased for control group employees and decreased for LIVE FOR LIFE participants. In contrast, salaried employees showed no significant intergroup differences in either 1980 or 1981.

Health Care Benefit Costs.   A companion economic study assessed the possible impact of LIVE FOR LIFE on the portion of health benefit costs for employees that were paid by Johnson & Johnson (Bly, Jones, & Richardson, 1986). Analysts studied the health care claims experience of all employees continuously employed from 1979 to 1983 (the study period) by three groups of Johnson & Johnson companies: (a) Those with no program, as of December 1983—the control group; (b) those who had the program in place for 18 to 30 months by that date; and (c) those with greater than 30 months of program experience as of that date. Data for subsequent periods are not available because the control group implemented the program, and assuring the quality of data from a new carrier was considered problematic. There were 5,192 employees in Group 1—LIFE FOR LIFE, 3,259 in Group 2—LIVE FOR LIFE, and 2,955 in Group 3—control. There were no work disruptions, such as strikes or layoffs, at any of these companies during the study period.

Table 11.5
Direct Economic Effects of LIVE FOR LIFE Program

Survey	Measure	Intervention groups	Control group	p-value
Impact on absenteeism (wage employees only)	**Unadjusted mean absentee hours**			
	Year 0 (baseline)	60.7	50.0	NR
	Year 1	65.5	64.5	NR
	Year 2	59.5	80.1	NR
	Adjusted mean absentee hours			
	Year 1	61.5	61.9	>0.1
	Year 2	56.5	76.5	<0.01
Impact on health care costs & utilization	**Mean annual inpatient cost increases in dollars, over 5 years**			
	LIVE FOR LIFE Group 1 (30-40 month program exposure)	$43.00	$76.00	<0.001
	LIVE FOR LIFE Group 2 (18-30 month program exposure)	$42.00	$76.00	<0.001
	Mean annual increment in hospital days per 1,000 employees, over 5 years			
	LIVE FOR LIFE Group 1	109.0	171.9	NS
	LIVE FOR LIFE Group 2	67.5	171.9	0.04

NS = Not significant.

NR = Not reported.

Note. From "Impact of Worksite Health Promotion on Health Care Costs and Utilization Evaluation of Johnson & Johnson's LIVE FOR LIFE Program" by J.L. Bly, R.C. Jones, and J.E. Richardson, 1986, *Journal of the American Medical Association,* **256**, pp. 3235-3240. Copyright 1986, American Medical Association. Adapted by permission. Also from "A Study of a Worksite Health Promotion Program and Absenteeism" by R.C. Jones, J.L. Bly, and J.E. Richardson, 1990, *Journal of Occupational Medicine,* **32**. Adapted by permission. Reprinted by permission.

Baseline intergroup differences in age, gender, job classification, location, and baseline health care utilization levels were observed and controlled through analysis of covariance. Inpatient costs for the two LIVE FOR LIFE groups grew at a significantly lower rate than did those for the control group, on average $43 and $42 a year for the study groups compared with $76 for the control group ($p < 0.001$; see Table 11.5). Intervention group costs in constant dollars approximately doubled during the 5-year study period, compared with the fourfold increase that occurred in costs of the control group. This difference equaled $245,079 (in 1979 dollars) a year for the LIVE FOR LIFE groups. Outpatient costs showed no significant difference between groups.

For both economic studies, observed differences between groups cannot be attributed solely to exposure to the LIVE FOR LIFE program. However, the very similar working environments of the intervention and control groups, coupled with statistical control for possible sources of bias, increases confidence that the program was likely to be the major explanatory variable.

Savings as a Result of Employee Health Promotion.   An estimate of savings from LIVE FOR LIFE was developed by combining economic data from the health benefits and absenteeism studies. LIVE FOR LIFE groups experienced additional health benefit expenses in the first 2 years, possibly the result of identification and medical follow-up of previously unknown health risks and other problems. However, the LIVE FOR LIFE groups achieved significant cost savings in the last 2 years of the study. During the fourth study year, companies that had LIVE FOR LIFE programs saved $223 per employee in 1990 dollars.

In the absenteeism study, after 2 years exposure to LIVE FOR LIFE, 20 hours per wage-earning employee per year were saved. The average wage employee earned $10 an hour in 1981 and $15.65 in 1990. In 1990 dollars, the 20-hour savings represents a net savings of $313 per employee per year. Because wage employees comprised approximately 50% of the total study population, the per-employee savings were estimated to be $156.50.

Assuming that savings held constant after the last year of the study, program savings from inpatient health care costs may have totaled $223.32 a year per employee by the fourth year after program implementation. Similarly, savings attributed to a reduction in absenteeism would total $156.50 a year per employee in the fifth year after program implementation.

Projected savings per employee in 1990 dollars (and achieved *after* programs have been in place for several years) are as follows:

Inpatient health care costs (achieved in the fourth year)	$223.32
Absenteeism reduction (for wage employees—achieved in the third year)	+ $156.50
Total savings	$379.82
Spending per employee on health promotion and fitness (1990 dollars)	− $225.00
Net savings per employee	$154.82
Benefit-to-cost ratio:	1.7:1.0

Any projections of future savings rely on several assumptions. However, given the observed pattern of increased effects over time both on health and on economic studies, the projection of ongoing benefits at the last level actually observed is a tenable action.

Indirect Economic Effects

Productivity, the domain with the most important potential economic impact, is also the most difficult to measure. Absenteeism is the most frequently assessed component, but other, softer measures may be of equal importance to employers in considering the return on their investment. Therefore, changes in employee attitudes, particularly those considered proxies for overall job satisfaction and commitment to the organization, were also assessed (Holzbach et al., 1990).

The epidemiological study of the four intervention and three control companies included six attitude scales in the baseline questionnaire and four single-item attitudinal measures. At the end of Year 1, and again at the end of Year 2, employees at both LIVE FOR LIFE and the control companies voluntarily completed the same questionnaire. Sample size and response rates at Year 0, Year 1, and Year 2, respectively, were (excluding those no longer employed at the LIVE FOR LIFE companies) 2,040 employees (77% responding), 1,223 (66%), and 1,551 (96%) in the LIVE FOR LIFE group, and 1,201 employees (70% responding), 764 (74%), and 796 (96%) in the control group. Of all those continuously employed individuals who responded at each data collection period, 63% were in LIVE FOR LIFE and 71% were controls. Scales ran from 0 (low) to 100 (high). (See Table 11.6 for participation rates.)

At Year 0, LIVE FOR LIFE employees had significantly higher scores for organizational commitment, relationships with coworkers, job satisfaction, and job security than did controls. LIVE FOR LIFE men were significantly younger than men in the control group, and LIVE FOR LIFE women held a significantly higher percentage of technical jobs than the control group. Although Year-2 volunteers and nonvolunteers for the first data

Table 11.6
Number of Participants and Participation Rates in Attitudinal Survey

Study year	LIVE FOR LIFE participants*	Controls
Year 0	2,040 (77%)	1,201 (70%)
Year 1	1,223 (66%)	764 (74%)
Year 2	1,551 (96%)	796 (96%)

*Excludes those not continuously employed at LIVE FOR LIFE companies during intervention period.

Note. From "Effect of a Comprehensive Health Promotion Program on Employee Attitudes" by R.L. Holzbach, P.V. Piserchia, D.W. McFadden, T.D. Hartwell, A.A. Herrmann, and J.E. Fielding, 1990, Journal of Occupational Medicine, 32. Reprinted by permission.

collection effort did not show significant differences on attitude measures, volunteers were younger than nonvolunteers and more likely to hold jobs paid on an hourly basis. All analyses were based on analysis of variance/covariance. Control variables were Year-0 score, age, gender, job classification, and Year-2 participation.

LIVE FOR LIFE companies showed significantly more positive changes overall at Years 1 and 2 in organizational commitment; satisfaction with supervision, working conditions, and pay and fringe benefits; and job security (see Table 11.7). Job competence saw an overall change from baseline, which was significant in Year 1 but not in Year 2. For most variables, the significant differences were due to increases in attitude scales among LIVE FOR LIFE employees and decreases among controls. The significant changes had occurred primarily in Year 1 and were maintained in Year 2. The observed positive effects on organizational commitment and satisfaction with working conditions occurred across all demographically defined subpopulations. Both participants and nonparticipants in formal LIVE FOR LIFE risk reduction programs had significantly more positive attitude-change scores on working conditions and job security at Year 2 compared to baseline scores than had control employees.

No overall differences in attitudinal changes were observed for job involvement, growth opportunities, respect from families and friends, and relations with coworkers. However, selected demographic subpopulations did show changes in some of these variables. Overall, the sustained effect over a broad range of attitude measures can be considered reflective of pervasive changes in the working environment due to program implementation.

Table 11.7
Indirect Economic Effects of the LIVE FOR LIFE Program

Measure	Adjusted least-squares means, after 2 years		p-value
	Intervention group	Control group	
Organizational commitment	79.3	75.8	<0.001
Job involvement	65.1	64.6	NS
Growth opportunities	63.5	62.6	NS
Supervision	67.2	64.1	<0.05
Working conditions	76.0	70.1	<0.001
Job competence	80.3	79.4	NS
Respect from family and friends	75.4	73.6	NS
Relations with coworkers	66.0	65.2	NS
Pay and fringe benefits	71.9	68.9	<0.01
Job security	72.1	69.6	<0.05

NS = Not significant.

Note. From "Effect of a Comprehensive Health Promotion Program on Employee Attitudes" by R.L. Holzbach, P.V. Piserchia, D.W. McFadden, T.D. Hartwell, A.A. Hermann, and J.E. Fielding, 1990, *Journal of Occupational Medicine,* **32**. Reprinted by permission.

Study Limitations

LIVE FOR LIFE has been subjected to more extensive evaluation than any other comprehensive worksite health promotion program. Nonetheless, the variety of studies are subject to common, study-specific limitations. The various individual investigations covered overlapping but different segments of the population for which the program was intended as well as different control groups, and different time periods were used during the 4 years overall that most of the published studies cover. Control groups were lost after several years because those companies were so impressed by the impact of LIVE FOR LIFE that they were unwilling to futher delay adopting the program. This occurred in much the same fashion that trials of a new drug tend to be abandoned as soon as a newer drug exhibits a significant advantage.

A problem common to all of the LIVE FOR LIFE studies is that a quasi-experimental design was employed, with nonrandom assignment to intervention and control conditions. In all studies, some differences between the groups were discerned at baseline. Although the studies use appropriate statistical methods to control for baseline differences in demographic, health, and other dependent variables of interest, systematic bias cannot be excluded as a contributor to the observed results. However, the fact that positive impacts were consistently observed for variables in both economic- and health-oriented studies increases confidence that the program caused the effects.

Although the effects observed are plausible, as one author stated "the mechanism by which an integrated, comprehensive, pervasive, and visible health promotion program can positively affect attitudes of both formal participating employees and those who only participate periodically in a health assessment are, nonetheless, conjectural and present an opportunity for additional research" (Holzbach et al., 1990, p. 978). The time frame and design did not permit assessment of impact on morbidity or mortality. We are thus unable to determine whether decreases in absenteeism or reductions in rate of health care costs are due to risk factor-associated conditions or a more general phenomenon. We do not know the relative contributions of general attitudinal changes versus risk factor changes to observed economic changes. Nor do we know whether attitudinal changes are independent of health risks. Do attitude changes precede, develop coincidently with, or follow lifestyle changes? Pursuing these and other questions will present a full research agenda for the future.

Implications for
Worksite Health Promotion Programs

LIVE FOR LIFE evaluation results suggest that a comprehensive worksite intervention can simultaneously affect a variety of employee behaviors and attitudes over 2 to 3 years. The observed differences are *conservative* estimates of the program's effects, because the control groups received repeated health profiles, a significant intervention which included both biometrics and considerable counseling by a trained nurse.

One of the important contributions of the LIVE FOR LIFE evaluations to the published literature is that almost all evaluations looked at the effects on the entire worksite population and were not limited to just those who volunteered to participate. LIVE FOR LIFE was conceived to have organization-wide effects, and it is therefore appropriate to consider effects on the employed population regardless of formal program participation. The effect of the program can be judged to be considerable, in contrast to the effects of many interventions that are measured on only a small subpopulation, for example, volunteers for a formal program component.

Because Johnson & Johnson interventions and related evaluations were not developed to test a specific theoretical construct, the mechanisms by which some results were achieved are still speculative. Results do suggest, however, that the mechanisms affect a range of outcome variables at differential rates. For example, significant effects on health risks were observed by the end of the first year. Significant economic impacts, including reduced absenteeism and inpatient utilization and costs, required 2 to 3 years. Positive effects on several work-related attitudes were consistently observed after 1 year of program exposure, but were further accentuated after 2 years.

Finally, the LIVE FOR LIFE experience, like that of other prospering worksite health promotion programs, strongly suggests that the largest benefits are paradoxically the most difficult to measure. Employee attitude survey results coupled with many anecdotes from employees and their managers point to enhanced productivity for both the individual and the organization. A shared perception of positive effects on productivity may account in part for the rapid growth in the prevalence and resources devoted to these activities, despite what some consider lack of definitive proof in dollar terms of a high return on investment.

Few corporations are prepared to invest the level of resources that Johnson & Johnson used to assess their program's effects. Additionally, the evaluation target moves as the program evolves. More flexibility makes it difficult to extrapolate results from a single model to the panoply of formats, delivery modes, and demographically diverse target populations. And because the worksite is the unit of analysis, a large number of worksites would have to be randomized to obtain sufficient statistical power for reasonable assumptions regarding the magnitude of program effects. This also is an improbability. It is rare today to find opportunities that allow isolation of the effects of a single program element, such as smoking cessation or fitness. Usually, we are left with a stew of multiple ingredients, seasoned for specific appetites, simmered for different lengths of time, and eaten in different settings. The growth of LIVE FOR LIFE and other programs suggest many hearty appetites for their benefits. And for the foreseeable future, the corpus of LIVE FOR LIFE studies is likely to remain the most comprehensive set of scientific studies of a comprehensive worksite health promotion program.

References

Blair, S.N., Piserchia, P.V., Wilbur, C.S., & Crowder, J.H. (1986). A public health intervention model for worksite health promotion: Impact on exercise and physical fitness in a health promotion plan after 24 months. *Journal of the American Medical Association*, **255**, 921-926.

Bly, J.L., Jones, R.C., & Richardson, J.E. (1986). Impact of worksite health promotion on health care costs and utilization. Evaluation of Johnson & Johnson's LIVE FOR LIFE program. *Journal of the American Medical Association*, **256**, 3235-3240.

Breslow, L., Fielding, J., Herrmann, A.A., & Wilbur, C.S. (1990). Worksite health promotion: Its evolution and the Johnson & Johnson experience. *Preventive Medicine, 19*, 13-21.

Holzbach, R.L., Piserchia, P.V., McFadden, D.W., Hartwell, T.D., Herrmann, A.A., & Fielding, J.E. (1990). Effect of a comprehensive health promotion program on employee attitudes. *Journal of Occupational Medicine, 32*, 973-978.

Jones, R.C., Bly, J.L., & Richardson, J.E. (1990). A study of a worksite health promotion program and absenteeism. *Journal of Occupational Medicine, 32*, 95-99.

Kornitzer, M., DeBacker, G., Dramaix, M., & Kittel, F. (1983). Belgian heart disease prevention project: Incidence and mortality results. *Lancet, 1*(8333), 1066-1070.

Maccoby, N., Farquhar, J.W., Wood, P.D., & Alexander, J. (1977). Reducing the risk of cardiovascular disease: Effects of a community-based campaign on knowledge and behavior. *Journal of Community Health, 3*, 100-114.

Multiple Risk Factor Intervention Trial (MRFIT) Research Group. (1982). Multiple risk factor intervention trial: Risk factor changes and mortality results. *Journal of the American Medical Association, 248*, 1465-1477.

National Center for Health Statistics. (1992). Advance report of final mortality statistics, 1989. *Monthly vital statistics report, 40*(8), Supplement 2. Hyattsville, MD: Public Health Service.

Salonen, J.T., Puska, P., Kottke, T.E., & Tuomilehto, J. (1981). Changes in smoking, serum cholesterol, and blood pressure levels during a community-based cardiovascular disease prevention program—The North Karelia project. *American Journal of Epidemiology, 144*, 81-94.

Settergren, S.K., Wilbur, C.S., Hartwell, T.D., & Rassweiler, J.H. (1983). Comparison of respondents and nonrespondents to a worksite health screen. *Journal of Occupational Medicine, 25*, 475-479.

Shipley, R.H., Orleans, C.T., Wilbur, C.S., Piserchia, P.V., & McFadden, D.W. (1988). Effect of the Johnson & Johnson LIVE FOR LIFE program on employee smoking. *Preventive Medicine, 17*, 25-34.

Weinstein, N.D., Grubb, P.D., & Vautier, J.S. (1986). Increasing automobile seat belt use: An intervention emphasizing risk susceptibility. *Journal of Applied Psychology, 71*, 285-290.

Wilbur, C.S., & Garner, D. (1984). Marketing health to employees, the Johnson & Johnson LIVE FOR LIFE program. In L.W. Frederiksen, L.J. Solomon, & K.A. Breheny (Eds.), *Marketing health behavior* (pp. 137-163). New York: Plenum.

Wilbur, C.S., Hartwell, T.D., & Piserchia, P.V. (1985). The Johnson & Johnson LIVE FOR LIFE program: Its organization and evaluation plan. In M. Cataldo & T. Coates (Eds.), *Health and industry: A behavioral medicine perspective* (pp. 338-350). New York: Wiley.

Appendix

Economic Impact
of Worksite Health Promotion

Joseph Opatz
David Chenoweth
Robert Kaman

Note. This paper, originally written in August 1991, is a summary of the Economic Impact of Worksite Health Promotion Conference held at the Texas College of Osteopathic Medicine, May 1990. Adapted by permission of Joseph Opatz, David Chenoweth, and Robert Kaman.

Panelists

The panelists at the conference whose proceedings and conclusions are summarized in this paper are

Robert L. Kaman, PhD, FAFB
Conference Chairman,
Texas College of Osteopathic Medicine

Joseph Opatz, PhD
Cochairman, St. Cloud State University

David Chenoweth, PhD, FAFB
Cochairman, East Carolina University

David Anderson, PhD
StayWell Health Management Systems, Inc.

William Baun, PhD, FAFB
Tenneco Corporation

Steven Blair, PED
Cooper Institute for Aerobics Research

Brenda Mitchell, PhD
Cooper Institute for Aerobics Research

Larry Gettman, PhD, FAFB
National Health Enhancement Systems

Richard Huset, MD
Health Decisions, Inc.

Robert Karch, EdD
American University

Roy Shephard, MD, PhD, DPE
University of Toronto

James Terborg, PhD
University of Oregon

Kenneth Warner, PhD
University of Michigan

Overview

The Association for Worksite Health Promotion has initiated a process to assess the economic impact of worksite health promotion programs. A panel of twelve leading researchers and practitioners working in this important area convened to address this issue. Along with 75 other participants at the conference, they worked to develop a consensus statement on the state of the art of the economic benefits of worksite health promotion. This commentary, summarized here, represents the association's continuing commitment in providing its membership and the greater business community with up-to-date information on worksite health promotion.

The authors conclude that economic benefits accrue from health promotion activities in the short term (less than five years). The long-term economic benefits of health promotion intervention and application in certain settings (such as small companies and primarily blue-collar organizations) remain less clear.

Introduction

Evolution of the Process

As health care costs continue to rise, and as American business is asked to assume a greater share of these costs, the focus has centered on strategies to contain these costs at the worksite (1-6). Long before the implementation of fiscal cost-containment efforts was initiated, companies began implementing worksite fitness programs for their employees (7). Generally developed as a demonstration of company support for improving the quality of life of employees, these programs seemed to create healthier, more productive employees as well. These original support programs evolved into enlarged health promotion programs, and documentation of their effectiveness became an area of interest for industry leaders. Cost-benefit and cost-effectiveness studies began to appear in literature, and the outcomes of these studies generally were positive (8-13). Worksite health promotion soon was proposed as a solution to increased health care costs (1), and as a result many American companies have created such programs.

Along with the proponents of these programs came the skeptics. Reviews of some of the program evaluations have suggested possibly compromised methodology (14, 63). In 1989, the Association for Worksite Health Promotion reviewed these program evaluations with the objective of summarizing all of the reported studies into a concise document valuable to both practitioners and managers alike. After reviewing the literature, the authors concluded that a consensus view is an elusive goal, since many of the program reports were inconclusive. Rather than a simple literature review, a more thorough analysis was required. A conference of the leading researchers and practitioners in the field was selected as the vehicle for this analysis. Solicitation of support for this project was rewarded by a generous grant of $10,000 from the Parke-Davis Company, the Texas College of Osteopathic Medicine in Fort Worth offered its facilities as host, and the association provided the logistics and staff support, enabling the conference to convene. The conference was held on May 19, 1990. This report summarizes the outcome.

Definition of Economic Impact of Health Promotion

1. *Measuring health promotion's effects.* The dollar savings inferred from the implementation of health promotion programs has been a primary focus for selling such programs to management (15, 16). Although the focus of this report is the economic benefits of health promotion, it must be remembered that other reasons exist for health promotion implementation (17-19). Public relations, marketing, employee benefits enhancement, and other reasons have motivated employers to implement worksite health promotion programs.

2. *Cost-benefit analysis.* Economic impact can be defined by two methods. The first is through the application of cost-benefit analysis, which is the process of assigning a dollar value to all costs associated with the program and assigning a dollar value to all benefits accrued as a result of the program. This can be shown in a simple ratio of benefits to cost, with any result greater than one indicating a positive benefit, and any less than one a negative benefit. While the equation is simple, the process of obtaining and inserting numbers can be most difficult. Several researchers (13, 20-23) have provided descriptions of the process of health promotion program cost-benefit analysis.

3. *Cost-effectiveness analysis.* The second method is cost-effectiveness analysis. Here we determine the dollar value of all costs of the program, then measure the benefits amassed in terms of some nonmonetary unit (such as extended life, quality of life, reduced risk factors, etc.). Cost-effectiveness analysis generally is used to compare different strategies for achieving a specific goal.

In order to obtain a complete cost-benefit or cost-effectiveness analysis, all actual and potential costs and benefits must be accounted for. In practice, this theoretical goal is rarely achieved. Instead, most studies focus on direct costs and benefits within a short time frame. Long-term benefits and costs, such as pensions and social security payments, are more difficult to assess. Several researchers have provided detailed descriptions of the process of health promotion program cost-effectiveness analysis (24-26), and others have discussed the differences between the two analytical strategies in detail (27-28).

Current Findings

Most of the research to date has focused on four* areas. The first to be considered, risk reduction, measures cost effectiveness (no specific dollar amount for the benefit is obtained). The next three allow for some measure of the savings in dollars accrued from health promotion, implementation (including absenteeism), productivity, and health care costs.

Risk Reduction or Behavior Change

Substantial evidence suggests that health promotion programs have an impact on risk reduction and behavioral change within employee groups. Such findings have been documented by evaluations of health promotion programs at Control Data (29), Johnson & Johnson (30-31), Blue Cross/ Blue Shield of Indiana (32-33), Canada Life Insurance Company (34), and NASA (35).
  Limitations:

- Lack of standardized measurement tools
- Inadequate control groups
- Not-at-risk levels represented

Health (Medical) Care Costs

Cost-benefit studies measuring medical care cost savings suggest positive benefits of health promotion to the employer. Since most studies reported thus far describe only relatively short-term evaluations and primarily measure direct, rather than indirect and long-term, costs of program implementation, more work will be required to firmly establish a positive cost-benefit relationship in this area.
  Substantial evidence suggests that risks are related to health care costs and that health promotion can reduce those risks. Studies have shown that health care utilization and their related costs are substantially less for health promotion participants than for nonparticipants over the short term. The Prudential Insurance Company (36), Kimberly-Clark (37), Blue

---

*A fifth area, turnover, is often cited as a measure of the impact of worksite health promotion, but the authors conclude that insufficient data exist thus far to determine if such programs have a positive economic impact.

Cross/Blue Shield of Indiana (32, 33), Johnson & Johnson (38), Control Data (29), Canada Life Insurance Company (34, 39), and Mesa Petroleum (12) have all documented such effects in their program evaluations.
Limitations:

- Small sample size
- Short observation periods
- Selection bias
- Data collection quality

Absenteeism

Exercise has been shown to have a positive effect on reducing absenteeism at the worksite. Fourteen of the approximately 20 studies reviewed (39) reported changes in absenteeism. Virtually all of these studies focus on the impact of exercise rather than broad health promotion programs on absenteeism. These studies consistently show one to two fewer absent days per year among participants. Virtually all of the studies published to date report consistently favorable results regardless of the methodology used. In a recent 2-year study conducted at 41 intervention and 19 control sites within the DuPont Corporation, disability-related absenteeism was reduced an average of 0.4 days per employee per year for health promotion program participants compared to control-group employees (62).
Limitations:

- Short periods of observation
- Inconsistent definitions of absenteeism
- Not differentiating between planned and unplanned absences
- Self-selection bias

Productivity

Substantial evidence suggests that the physical fitness component of health promotion has an impact on improving worker productivity (generally measured in cost-effectiveness rather than cost-benefit terms). Productivity may be defined as what a person produces while at work. This can be both physical and mental output. Many studies show that fit and healthy employees obtain higher performance ratings than those in lower fitness categories (40, 41). Research evidence suggests that fit individuals have fewer injuries (42), can perform at a higher level on the job (43, 44), and return to the job quicker than less fit individuals following an injury (45, 46).

Studies measuring psychological change as a benefit of worksite health promotion also demonstrate positive benefits on worker productivity (47). Studies of EAP-related programs (48-52), stress management (53), and other mental health programs associated with health promotion demonstrate the benefit of early intervention on productivity and psychological health. These programs also appear to help protect the company from diminished worker productivity in the future. In general, studies have not addressed the question of financial savings associated with improved worker productivity as a result of implementing worksite health promotion programs.

Limitations:

- Few worksite programs evaluated
- Nonstandardized measures of productivity
- Inadequate control groups
- Short observation periods

Computer Simulation

The prospect of developing valid computer simulations of the costs, benefits, and effectiveness of worksite health promotion programs is promising. By creating well-designed computer models into which an organization can input its specific data (such as health promotion program costs, health care costs, absenteeism records, etc.), estimates of the impact of their health promotion efforts can be determined without a substantial investment in research and program evaluation. To date, the small but significant number of published studies generally project benefits greater than costs, within the varying parameters generated by sensitivity analysis (57-61). Computer simulation can be a cost-effective method of projecting the benefits of health promotion by providing otherwise unavailable information to management in the process of deciding to implement or sustain a program.

Summary of Findings

Table 1
Strength of Relationships

Area studies	Potential economic impact of health promotion	
	Short-term	Long-term
Absenteeism	Moderate to strong	Inconclusive
Employee health behavior	Moderate	Inconclusive
Health care costs	Moderate	Inconclusive
Productivity	Moderate to strong	Inconclusive
Computer simulation*	Promising	Inconclusive

*As an evaluation method.

Further Considerations

Continued study is needed to confirm that a positive impact of worksite health promotion, as most studies to date suggest, does indeed occur. These studies should address the following issues:

1. Generalizability: Manufacturing and insurance companies have been studied most often. Other industry programs should be evaluated as well.
2. Employee population issues: Most studies have focused on male-dominated, white-collar employee groups. Minority and blue-collar workers also should be studied.
3. Organizational size issues: Most organizations studied thus far have been large. The impact of worksite health promotion programs in small company settings also must be evaluated.
4. Outcome of economic impact studies: Renewed emphasis should be placed on studies of cost-effectiveness rather than cost benefit, until the methodology is developed for obtaining accurate and comprehensive long-term dollar estimates of benefits (and costs).
5. Research design: Many worksite evaluations use quasi-experimental designs, which may allow selection bias, premeasurement sensitivity, multiple intervention interference, and other factors of uncertainty. Future studies should be designed to minimize these limitations.

Conclusions

Efforts to assess the economic benefits of health promotion at the worksite have been undertaken for little more than a decade. Despite the relative infancy of the field of health promotion evaluation, significant gains have been made in understanding the nature of the impact of health promotion as a cost-savings strategy. Much of the early initiative to implement health promotion at the worksite was based on the assumption that such initiatives would ultimately lead to financial savings. This assumption was based on the premise that by changing individual employee behavior (such as reducing the incidence of smoking), the risks of disease and death associated with these factors would also be reduced; an extension of that assumption was the further assumption that such risk reduction would ultimately lead to savings in the areas of health care costs, absenteeism, turnover, and productivity.

To date, there is evidence that well-designed and carefully targeted health promotion programs can cause changes in employee behavior and reduce associated risk factors. Although reported cost savings may not be as substantial as behavioral and risk reduction changes, numerous health promotion programs have reported economic benefits. Of the studies conducted to measure financial impact, most have focused on the cost-effectiveness (nonmonetized) benefits of health promotion. These studies have *all* shown positive outcomes. Those few studies performed to date on the cost benefits (monetizing both costs and benefits) of health promotion strongly suggest a positive financial impact. Because of the natural limitations imposed on studies regarding behavior measurement and the small number of studies available, more rigorous study is needed to clarify and understand the long-term economic impact of worksite health promotion programs.

Acknowledgments

The Economic Impact of Worksite Health Promotion Conference was supported by a grant from the Parke-Davis Company, Ann Arbor, Michigan. Additional support for the conference was provided by the Texas College of Osteopathic Medicine. This document was printed through the generosity of CIGNA Corporation.

References

1. Herzlinger, R.E.; Calkins, D. How companies tackle health care costs. Part III. *Harvard Business Review*, pp 70-80, January-February 1986.
2. Gray, H.J. The role of business in health promotion: a brief overview. *Preventive Medicine*, 12:654-657; 1983.
3. Demkovich, L.E. Business, as a health care consumer, is paying heed to the bottom line. *National Journal*, pp 851-854, April 24, 1980.
4. Elias, W.S.; Murphy, R.J. The case for health promotion programs containing health care costs: a review of the literature. *The American Journal of Occupational Therapy*, 40(11): 759-763; 1986.
5. McCoy, J. Wellness program can be a cost effective solution to soaring health care costs. *American Journal of Compensation and Benefits*, 278-284; March-April 1988.
6. Shephard, R.J. The impact of exercise upon medical costs. *Sports Medicine*, 2:133-143, 1985.
7. Conrad, C.C. A chronology of the development of corporate fitness in the United States. *Fitness in Business*, 1(5):156-166; 1987.
8. Kaman, R.L. Costs and benefits of corporate health promotion. *Fitness in Business*, 2(2):39-44; 1987.
9. Grana, J. Weighing the costs and benefits of worksite health promotion. *Corporate Comment*, 1(5): 18-29; 1985.

10. Chenoweth, D. Health promotion: benefit vs. costs. *Occupational Health and Safety*, 37-41; 1983.
11. Ostwald, S.K. Cost benefit analysis: a framework for evaluating corporate health promotion programs. *American Association of Occupational Health Nurses Journal*, 34(8): 377-382; 1986.
12. Gettman, L.R. Cost/benefit analysis of a corporate fitness program. *Fitness in Business*, 1(1):11-17; 1986.
13. Opatz, J. Health promotion evaluation: measuring the organizational impact. Stevens Point, WI: National Wellness Institute; 1987:1-13.
14. Warner, K.E.; Wickizer, T.M.; Wolfe, R.A.; Schildroth, J.E.; Samuelson, M.H. Economic implications of workplace health promotion programs: review of the literature. *Journal of Occupational Medicine*, 30(2):106-112; 1988.
15. Kaman, R.L.; Huckaby, J. Justification of employee fitness programs: cost vs. benefit. *Fitness in Business*, 3(3):90-95; 1988.
16. Jose, W.S.; Anderson, D.R.; Haight, S.A. The StayWell strategy for health care cost containment. In: Opatz, J., ed. Health Promotion Evaluation: Measuring the organizational impact. Stevens Point, WI: National Wellness Institute; 1987: p. 15-34.
17. Walsh, D.C.; Egdahl, R.H. Corporate perspectives on worksite wellness programs: a report on the seventh Pew Fellows conference. *Journal of Occupational Medicine*, 31(6):551-556; 1989.
18. Warner, K.E. Selling health promotion to corporate America: uses and abuses of the economic argument. *Health Education Quarterly*, 14(1):39-55; 1987.
19. Blair, S.N.; Piserchia, P.V.; Wilbur, C.S.; Crowder, J.H. A public health intervention model for worksite health promotion. *Journal of the American Medical Association*, 255(7):921-926; 1986.
20. Murphy, R.J.; Elias, W.S.; Gasparotto, G.; Huset, R.A. Cost-benefit analysis in worksite health promotion evaluation. *Fitness in Business*, 1(5):15-19; 1987.
21. Smith, K.J. A framework for appraising corporate wellness investments. *Internal Auditor*, pp 28-33, December 1987.
22. Jones, L.; Baker, M.R. The application of health economics to health promotion. *Community Medicine*, 8(3):224-229; 1986.
23. Chenoweth, D. Nurses's intervention in specific risk factors in high risk employees. *American Association of Occupational Health Nursing Journal*, 37(9):367-373; 1989.
24. Banta, H.D.; Luce, B.R. Assessing the cost-effectiveness of prevention. *Journal of Community Health*, 9(2):145-165; 1983.
25. Fielding, J.E. Effectiveness of employee health improvement programs. *Journal of Occupational Medicine*, 24(11):907-916; 1982.
26. Bertera, R.L.; Oehl, L.K.; Telepchak, J.M. Self-help versus group approaches to smoking cessation in the workplace: eighteen-month

follow-up and cost analysis. *American Journal of Health Promotion*, 4(3):187-192; 1990.

27. Rogers, P.J.; Eaton, E.K.; Bruhn, J.G. Is health promotion cost effective? *Preventive Medicine*, 10:324-339; 1981.

28. DeFriese, G.H.; Barry, P.Z. Questions about costs, benefits, and the effectiveness of health promotion programs. *Mobius*, 2(3):142-146; 1982.

29. Anderson, D.R.; Jose, W.S. Employee lifestyle and the bottom line. *Fitness in Business*, 2(3):86-91; 1987.

30. Shipley, R.H.; Orleans, C.T.; Wilbur, C.S.; Piserchia, P.V.; McFadden, D.W. Effect of the Johnson & Johnson LIVE FOR LIFE Program on employee smoking. *Preventive Medicine*, 17:25-34; 1988.

31. Wilbur, C.S. The Johnson & Johnson Program. *Preventive Medicine*, 12:672-681; 1983.

32. Gibbs, J.O.; Mulvaney, D.; Henes, C.; Reed, R.W. Worksite health promotion: five-year trend in employee health care costs. *Journal of Occupational Medicine*, 27:826-830; 1985.

33. Mulvaney, D.E.; Gibbs, J.O.; Reed, W.R.; Grove, D.A.; Skinner, T.W. Staying alive and well at Blue Cross and Blue Shield of Indiana. In Opatz, J.P., ed. Health Promotion Evaluation: Measuring the Organizational Impact. Stevens Point, WI: National Wellness Institute; 1987: p. 131-141.

34. Shephard, R.J.; Corey, P.; Cos, M.H. Health hazard appraisal—the influence of an employee fitness programme. *Canadian Journal of Public Health*, 73:183-187; 1982.

35. Durbeck, D.C.; Heinzelmann, F.; Schacter, J. The National Aeronautics and Space Administration—U.S. Public Health Service Health evaluation and enhancement program. *The American Journal of Cardiology*, 30:784-790; 1972.

36. Brown, D.W.; Russell, M.L.; Morgan, J.L.; Optenberg, S.A.; Clarke, A.E. Reduced disability and health care costs in an industrial fitness program. *Journal of Occupational Medicine*, 26:809-815; 1984.

37. Berry, C.A. *An approach to good health for employees and reduced health care costs for industry*. Health Insurance Association of America, p 9, 1981.

38. Bly, J.; Jones, R.C.; Richardson, R.E. Impact of worksite health promotion on health care costs and utilization. *Journal of the American Medical Association*, 256:3235-3240; 1986.

39. Shephard, R.J. Current perspectives on the economics of fitness and sport with particular reference to worksite programs. *Sports Medicine*, 7:286-389; 1989.

40. Bernacki, E.J.; Baun, W.B. The relationship of job performance to exercise adherence in a corporate fitness program. *Journal of Occupational Medicine*, 26(7):529-531; 1984.

41. Pender, N.J.; Smith, L.C.; Vernoff, J.A. Building better workers. *American Association of Occupational Health Nurses Journal*, 35(9):386-390; 1987.
42. Tsai, S.P.; Bernacki, E.J.; Baun, W.B. Injury prevalence and associated costs among participants of an employee fitness program. *Preventive Medicine*, 17(4):475-482; 1988.
43. Shephard, R.J.; Cox, M.; Corey, P. Fitness program participation: its effects on worker performance. *Journal of Occupational Medicine*, 23:359-363; 1981.
44. Rhodes, E.C.; Dunwoody, D. Physiological and attitudinal changes of individuals involved in an employee fitness program. *Canadian Journal of Public Health*, 71:331-336; 1980.
45. Cristina, J. GTE: Florida's in-house physical therapy program. *Corporate Fitness*, 65-67; September 1987.
46. Fitzler, S.L.; Berger, R.A. Chelsea back program: one year later. *Occupational Health and Safety*, 52(7):52-54; 1983.
47. Rudman, W.J. Do onsite health and fitness programs affect worker productivity? *Fitness in Business*, 2(1):2-8; 1987.
48. Bensinger, A.; Pilkington, C. An alternate method in the treatment of alcoholism: The United Technologies corporation day treatment program. *Journal of Occupational Medicine*, 300-303; 1983.
49. Blum, T.; Roman, R. Alcohol, drugs, and EAPs: new data from a national study. *The Almacan*, 16:20-23; 1986.
50. McGaffey, T.N. New horizons in organizational stress prevention approaches. *Personnel Administrator*, 11:26-32; 1978.
51. Norris, E. Alcohol: companies are learning it pays to help workers beat the bottle. *Business Insurance*, November 16, 1981.
52. Schrier, J.W. A survey on drug abuse in organizations. *Personnel Journal*, pp 478-484; 1983.
53. Manuso, J.S.J. The Equitable Life Assurance Society program. *Preventive Medicine*, 12:658-662; 1983.
54. Eggum, I.R.; Keller, P.J.; Burton, W.N. Nurse/health counseling model for a successful alcohol assistance program. *Journal of Occupational Medicine*, 22(8):545-548; 1980.
55. Rosen, R. Healthy companies: a human resources approach. New York: AMA Membership Publication Division; 1986.
56. Jaffee, D.; Scott, C.; Orioli, E. Stress management: programs and prospects. *American Journal of Health Promotion*, 1:29-37; 1986.
57. Terborg, J.R. Cost benefit analysis of the Adolph Coors Wellness Program. Copyrighted, unpublished report, College of Business Administration, University of Oregon, Eugene, OR; December 1988.
58. Hatziandreu, E.I.; Kopland, J.P.; Weinstein, M.C.; Caspersen, C.J.; Warner, K.E. A cost-effectiveness analysis of exercise as a health promotion activity. *American Journal of Public Health*, 78(11):1417-1421; 1988.

59. Keeler, E.B.; Manning, W.G.; Newhouse, J.P.; Sloss, E.M.; Wasserman, J. The external costs of a sedentary lifestyle. *American Journal of Public Health*, 79(8):975-981; 1989.
60. Huset, R. Tying your program to the bottom line. *Health Action Managers*, pp 6-9; April 25, 1988.
61. Murphy, R.J.; Elias, W.S.; Gasparotto, G.; Huset, R. Cost-benefit analysis in worksite health promotion evaluation. *Fitness in Business*, 2(1):15-19; 1987.
62. Bertera, R.L. The effects of workplace health promotion on absenteeism and employment costs in a large industrial population. *American Journal of Public Health*, 80(9):1101-1105; 1990.
63. Terborg, J. Health promotion at the worksite: a research challenge for personnel and human resources management. *Research in Personnel and Human Resources Management*, 4:225-267; 1986.
64. Tsai, P.T.; Bernacki, E.J.; Lucas, L.J. A longitudinal method of evaluating employee turnover. *Journal of Business and Psychology*, 3(4):465-473; 1989.
65. Tsai, P.T.; Baun, W.B.; Bernacki, E.J. Relationship of employee turnover to exercise adherence in a corporate fitness program. *Journal of Occupational Medicine*, 29(7):572-575; 1987.

Index

About the Authors

Joseph P. Opatz, PhD, is an administrator and adjunct professor at St. Cloud State University as well as a state legislator in the Minnesota House of Representatives. He is the author of *A Primer of Health Promotion: Creating Healthy Organizational Cultures* and the editor and coauthor of *Health Promotion Evaluation: Measuring the Organizational Impact*. He has also served as a founding editor of *The American Journal of Health Promotion* and was the founder of the National Wellness Association.

Opatz has been active in the field of wellness and health promotion since 1980, assisting numerous corporations, hospitals, schools, and other institutions in establishing health promotion programs. He is an active member of the Association for Worksite Health Promotion and held the office of First Vice President for Special Projects from 1990 through 1992. He earned his PhD in education from the University of Minnesota in 1982.

John P. Allegrante, PhD, is an associate professor of health education and chairman of the Department of Health and Nutrition Education at Teachers College and an associate professor of clinical public health in sociomedical sciences at the School of Public Health, Columbia University, where he has been a member of the faculty since 1979. He was a W.K. Kellogg Foundation Fellow from 1985 to 1988 and a Pew Health Policy Fellow at the RAND/UCLA Center for Health Policy Study during 1987 and 1988. He is a coauthor, with Richard P. Sloan and Jessie C. Gruman, of *Investing in Employee Health: A Guide to Effective Health Promotion at the Worksite* (Jossey-Bass, 1987) and is a frequent conference speaker on issues in worksite health promotion.

David Anderson, PhD, is vice-president of operations for StayWell Health Management Systems, a leading national provider of wellness and employee assistance programs headquartered in Eagan, Minnesota. He has worked in the health management field since 1979, focusing primarily on program development and evaluation. During this period, he directed the 10-year StayWell program evaluation, which is recognized as a milestone in establishing the cost impact of worksite wellness. Anderson has published 20 articles and spoken at more than 50 national and regional conferences on wellness and health care cost management. He is also the editor of the DataBase section of the *American Journal of Health Promotion*, the leading research journal in the health promotion field. Before joining StayWell, Anderson spent 5 years as a consultant designing and evaluating innovative health benefit strategies. Before his full-time involvement in health management, he was on the psychology faculty at the University of Wisconsin-Stevens Point. Anderson holds a PhD in psychology and is a licensed consulting psychologist.

Kathleen C. Brown, RN, PhD, is a professor and director of occupational health nursing at the University of Alabama School of Nursing, Birmingham.

David Chenoweth, PhD, FAWHP, is a professor and director of the Worksite Health Promotion Studies program at East Carolina University, Greenville, North Carolina. He is the author of several books, including *Planning Health Promotion at the Worksite* and *Health Care Cost Management: Strategies for Employers* published by Brown & Benchmark. For over a decade he has been president of Health Management Associates, a consulting firm specializing in health care cost management and health care data analysis services for businesses and industries. Since 1988 he has chaired the Business and Industry committee within the North Carolina Governor's Council on Physical Fitness and Health.

Jonathan E. Fielding, MD, MPH, MBA, is vice-president and health director responsible for scientific affairs and research at Johnson & Johnson Health Management, Inc. He also serves as vice-president, Health Policy Analysis and Planning, at Johnson & Johnson. He holds graduate degrees in medicine and public health from Harvard University and an MBA in finance from Wharton School of Business. He is a fellow of the American Academy of Pediatrics and the American College of Preventive Medicine. He is also professor of public health and pediatrics at UCLA's Schools of Public Health and Medicine where he teaches courses in organization, delivery, and financing of health care in the United States. His current research interests include the effectiveness of disease prevention and health promotion programs and private sector support for health system reform.

Kristan D. Goldfein, EdD, received her doctoral degree in health education from Teachers College, Columbia University. Since 1991, she has been coordinating health promotion programs at the Morgan Guaranty Trust Company in New York City. She is a member of the National Wellness Association and is on the Worksite Advisory Board of the March of Dimes New York Division.

Lawrence W. Green, DrPH, is director of the Institute of Health Promotion Research, a professor of health care and epidemiology, and head of the Division of Preventive Medicine and Health Promotion at the University of British Columbia. He was formerly vice-president and director of the health promotion program for the Kaiser Family Foundation. He was founding director of the Center for Health Promotion Research and Development at the University of Texas Health Science Center in Houston and of the graduate program in health education at Johns Hopkins University. He served the Carter administration as director of the U.S. Office of Health Promotion.

Jeffrey S. Harris, MD, MPH, MBA, is a principal and Western Regional Practice Leader for the Alexander & Alexander Consulting Group's Health Strategies unit. As such he manages client projects in strategic health and workers' compensation management, including data analysis, program strategy and design, vendor evaluation, operational analysis, and quality improvement. He also develops new products and marketing concepts. Previously he served as a corporate director of health care management, a public health official, an HMO medical director, and was in the private practice of occupational, preventive, family, and emergency medicine. He is coauthor and editor of *Managing Employee Health Care Costs: Assuring Quality and Value*, *The OEM Health and Safety Manual*, *Health Promotion in the Workplace*, and the upcoming volumes *Strategic Health Management* and *Reinventing Medicine: The Case for Total Quality Improvement*. He has also written many journal articles, video scripts, and health education materials. He speaks often at national and regional conferences. He is a recreational athlete, musician, gardener, and father of five and is married to a health care attorney and musician.

James C. Hilyer, EdD, MPH, is an instructor at the University of Alabama School of Medicine (Birmingham) and director of the fitness center for the city of Birmingham.

Steve Hoover, PhD, is an associate professor in the Department of Applied Psychology at St. Cloud State University, St. Cloud, Minnesota. He is currently serving as Interim Assistant Dean for the College of Education at St. Cloud State. His areas of interest include program evaluation designs, cognition and instruction, and the factors involved in problem solving and problem-finding behavior.

Marilyn Jensen, PhD, is a professor in the Department of Applied Psychology at St. Cloud State University, St. Cloud, Minnesota. She serves as co-coordinator of the Chemical Dependency Training Program and is interested in prevention, treatment, and training issues in the addictions field. Her research has addressed ethical issues for addiction professionals and has included analysis of the relationship between substance abuse and health behaviors. She is currently investigating variables controlling gambling behavior.

William S. Jose, PhD, is an associate professor and director of research at Northwestern College of Chiropractic, Bloomington, Minnesota. He is also president of OverView Consulting, through which he pursues his interest in worksite health promotion and risk-rated benefit plans. He received his PhD in quantitative social psychology from Stanford University and was a postdoctoral fellow at the M.S. Hershey Medical Center, Pennsylvania State University College of Medicine. He worked for 8 years with the StayWell health promotion program at Control Data Corporation. He is widely published in the health promotion field and has a particular interest in incentives for risk reduction in the worksite. He is also a contributing editor for the *American Journal of Health Promotion*. In 1989 he was honored with the Outstanding Research Award from the National Wellness Institute.

Robert Kaman, PhD, is an associate professor in public health/preventive medicine and physiology at the Texas College of Osteopathic Medicine. He received his master's and doctoral degrees in biochemistry and nutrition from Virginia Tech. Kaman has researched the effects of diet and exercise on metabolism and performance and the economics of employee health promotion. He is an active member of the Association of Worksite Health Promotion, American College of Sports Medicine, and American Public Health Association and past-president of the Association for Fitness in Business.

Robert C. Karch, EdD, is the executive director and founder of the National Center for Health Fitness and is one of the nation's foremost authorities on the development and promotion of health and fitness programs. In addition to his professorial appointment at American University, he has served as a consultant to numerous businesses and government agencies. He has received numerous awards and honors, including the U.S. Jaycees Healthy American Fitness Leader's Award, and has published and presented a wide range of health and fitness issues.

Chris Y. Lovato, PhD, is an associate professor in the Graduate School of Public Health, and codirector of the Center for Behavioral and Community Health Studies at San Diego State University. She was formerly director of health promotion for Student Health Services at San Diego State University and was a research assistant professor at the Center for Health Promotion Research and Development, University of Texas Health Science Center at Houston. She is currently conducting research in the areas of HIV prevention among college youth and community health promotion programs for Hispanic populations. She previously served as principal investigator to evaluate a worksite health promotion program for union-based workers.

Wendy D. Lynch, PhD, is a principal with Health Decisions, Inc., in Evergreen, CO, and is affiliated with the University of Colorado Health Sciences Center in Denver. She has served as an evaluation consultant for several large corporations nationwide. Her research and publications have focused on the impact of health promotion programs and measurement issues regarding the evaluation of cost-containment interventions. Lynch has a personal and professional interest in the benefits of exercise, and she takes advantage of the many sport and recreation activities available in Colorado.

Robert Murphy received his PhD in experimental and physiological psychology from the University of Tennessee and has been a postdoctoral fellow in cardiovascular health behavior in the Department of Epidemiology, University of Minnesota. He is currently chair and professor of the Department of Applied Psychology, a research associate and advisory board member of the Human Performance Laboratory, and codirector of the Center for Lifestyle Enhancement at St. Cloud State University. In addition, he is a licensed psychologist in the state of Minnesota. He is currently teaching, publishing, and consulting in the areas of health psychology, behavioral medicine, behavior therapy, and program evaluation.

Todd Rogers, PhD, is a senior research scientist at the Stanford University School of Medicine and director of the Health Promotion Resource Center within the Stanford Center for Research in Disease Prevention. He received his degree in clinical psychology from Pennsylvania State University and completed postdoctoral training in epidemiology and prevention with the Stanford Heart Disease Prevention Program. His research has focused on the application of community development approaches to complex culturally-based problems such as chronic disease, and alcohol, tobacco, and other drug abuse. He has provided technical assistance and training on community-directed health promotion to dozens of public and private health agencies at the local, state, and federal levels and serves on a variety of professional advisory panels and public service committees.

Marc A. Schaeffer, PhD, is the associate director of research of the National Center for Health Fitness and a research assistant professor at American University. With his primary interests in applied research methodology and data analysis, he has published articles dealing with worksite health promotion evaluation and the relationship between behavior and disease.

William J. Schneider, MD, MPH, is a graduate of Tufts University, the Columbia University College of Physicians and Surgeons, and the Columbia University School of Public Health. After completing his postgraduate medical training in internal medicine and infectious diseases at the University of Chicago, the New York Hospital, and New York University Medical Center, he held hospital and faculty appointments at New York University and the Albert Einstein College of Medicine. In 1981 he joined the staff of the Morgan Guaranty Trust Company where he is presently Director of Health Services. He remains on the faculty of the Albert Einstein College of Medicine. He is an officer of the American College of Occupational and Environmental Medicine and a member of several other local and national organizations in medicine, occupational medicine, and infectious diseases.

Anastasia M. Snelling, PhD, is the associate director of operations for the National Center for Health Fitness and holds adjunct professor appointments at American University and George Washington University. Her interests deal with the role of nutrition education in health promotion and the education of leaders in the field of health promotion. She is also very active in a number of professional societies, including the Association for Worksite Health Promotion and the Society for Nutrition Education.

Gene L. Stainbrook, PhD, MPH, is a research analyst and planner with the Maternal Child Health Program of the Oregon Health Division. He was formerly a faculty associate at the Center for Health Promotion Research and Development at the University of Texas Health Sciences Center in Houston.

Maura O. Stevenson, PhD, formerly the associate director of programs at the National Center for Health Fitness, is an adjunct faculty member at American University where she teaches in the graduate program of the Department of Health and Fitness, and at the Carrol Community College of Westminster, Maryland, where she teaches health and life fitness. Her areas of expertise include worksite health promotion, cardiac rehabilitation, and graded exercise testing.

Kenneth A. Theriault, MBA, is a senior consultant of methodology and analysis design for Corporate Health Strategies in New Haven, Connecticut. He was previously a senior consultant with the Alexander & Alexander Consulting Group, where he was responsible for data analysis and consulting in the areas of medical cost management and quality assurance. His consulting activities include managed care evaluation, strategic health care planning, managed fee-for-service consulting, and evaluating employee assistance and health promotion programs. Theriault has also served as Associate Director, Clinical Information Service, for Yale-New Haven Hospital. He holds a BS in Administrative Science and an MDiv from Yale University. His MBA in Health Care Administration is from Sacred Heart University.

R. William Whitmer, MBA, is founder, president, and CEO of Wellness South, Inc. As such he has directed the design, development, marketing, and production of comprehensive health promotion programs for over 75 clients including Coca-Cola, Uniroyal, the City of Birmingham, South Central Bell, and Dresser Industries, Inc. He is author of *Whitmer's Guide to Total Wellness* and a contributor to the scientific literature. A frequent speaker at national health promotion conferences, he is a competitive runner who regularly competes in the New York City, Marine Corps, and other marathons.

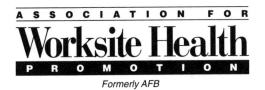

MEMBERSHIP FACT SHEET

AWHP Membership Benefits

Individual members and the official representatives for company memberships receive these "tangible" benefits:

- A subscription to the *American Journal of Health Promotion*
- A subscription to the AWHP *Action* newsletter
- The annual Who's Who Membership Directory and Resource Guide (an exclusive benefit) and free inclusion if membership status is current as of January 1
- Automatic membership in regional and local sections
- Eligibility to subscribe to the JOB Opportunity Bureau (an exclusive benefit)
- Preferred rates for the AWHP conference and events

In addition, the Association will offer and arrange special programs or services for AWHP members only.

Associate member companies receive the following additional benefits:

- Eligibility to exhibit at the Annual Conference
- Preferred rate (an additional 10% reduction of the low member price) on mailing list rental
- Preferred rate (10% reduction) on all advertising rates in AWHP publications

AWHP Membership Categories

The association has a category of membership available to meet your situation. Following is a listing of the types of memberships provided. Please note that only the Professional Member has the right to hold office or vote on Association matters.

1. **Individual Memberships.** These memberships are in the name of the individual rather than the company or organization. Transfers of individual memberships may only be done with the expressed permission of the original holder of the membership.

   A. **Professional Member** is for individuals who derive income from a health promotion profession by providing educational development, management services, or evaluations of health promotion programs.

   B. **General Member** is for individuals who have an active interest in health promotion, but do not derive income from a health promotion profession.

   C. **Student Member** is for full-time undergraduate and graduate students enrolled in a program of study related to health promotion. (AWHP also provides a student chapter program at qualified institutions. Please call the AWHP office for more information.)

2. **Company Memberships.** These memberships are in the name of a firm, business, or organization. The company/organization designates the person or persons who will represent them with the Association and pays annual dues for each representative. Memberships may be transferred by the company/organization upon written notice to AWHP.

  A. **Associate Member** is available to any firm, business, or corporation engaged in selling products or services to members of the Association.

  B. **Company/Organization Member** is available to any firm, business, not-for-profit organization, or institution with an active interest in health promotion or that may be helpful in carrying out the objectives of the Association.

AWHP Application for Membership
(Please type, print, or attach a business card)

Date of Application _____ Name _____ Nickname _____
                                      (First)   (M.I.)   (Last)

Title _____ Company/Organization _____

Address _____ City _____ State _____ Zip _____

Phone (_____) _____ Fax (_____) _____

> Please check the membership you are applying for and submit the appropriate annual fee in U.S. dollars or the equivalent. (Memberships are based on the calendar year. Pay the full amount for the first year to activate your membership. The second year will be prorated according to when you joined.)

❑ Professional Member — $130   ❑ Associate Member — $350

❑ General Member — $130   ❑ Student Member* — $70

❑ Company/Organization Member — $250

*A student application must be accompanied by a letter from the registrar's office or a current transcript.

❑ Check enclosed for $ _____ ❑ Bill me for $ _____

❑ Charge $ _____ to my ❑ Visa ❑ MasterCard Acct. # _____

Exp. Date _____ Signature _____

Sponsor's name/who introduced you to AWHP _____
                                                            (Optional)

**You will begin receiving services upon receipt of payment.
Please allow 4–6 weeks for initial receipt of publication.**

**If you have any questions regarding your membership services,
please call AWHP at (708)480-9574, fax (708)480-9282.**

Mail completed application to AWHP, 60 Revere Dr., Ste. 500, Northbrook, IL 60062.

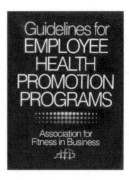